A Clinical Manual of Practical Oriental Medicine

Breakthrough: Integrated Synergy Therapeutics
Volume 1, Revision

Masaaki Nakano, DOM

Mateo Bernal, DOM

Disclaimer:

The information provided in this book is for general medical education purposes only, does not claim any medical benefits, and does not claim to cure any disease or medical condition. The information is not warranted to be inclusive of all approaches to a medical issue or exclusive of other methods for obtaining the same result. The material is not meant to substitute for the independent professional judgment of a physician or other health care professional relative to diagnostic and treatment options for a specific patient's medical condition. Masaaki Nakano, DOM does not warrant the completeness, accuracy, or usefulness of any opinions, options, advice, services, or other information provided through this book. In no event the author, co-author, publisher, and agents are not liable for any damages arising from or in connection with the use of or the reliance on any information in this book or DVD. Always consult a licensed medical professional before beginning or using any of the methods disclosed in this treatise.

The material in this book may not be reproduced or transmitted in whole or in part in any medium. This includes and is not limited to any electronic, or other physical, or cyber medium. You must have the express written authorization of the publisher and Dr. Masaaki Nakano. To request authorization, please contact Dr. Nakano describing the particular material to use, how you will use it, the purpose of the use and the number of copies that will be used. You can contact Dr. Nakano at drnakanoist@gmail.com

Copyright © 2013 Masaaki Nakano

1st Revision. 09-03-2014. All rights reserved.

ISBN-13: 9781492320661

CONTENTS

FOREWARD   3

PREFACE   5

INTEGRATED SYNERGY THERAPEUTICS   8

SIMILARITIES AND DIFFERENCES BETWEEN IST AND TCM   10

PRACTICAL ACU-ZONE THERAPY   12

THEORY   15
- DEFINITION OF A ZONE   15
- WHAT IS DISEASE? WHAT IS HEALTH?   15
- ACUPUNCTURE AND CHANNEL THEORY   17
- CONCEPT OF SYNERGETIC QI   18
- TOOLS/ACUPUNCTURE TECHNIQUE   19

DIAGNOSIS   20
- PALPATORY DIAGNOSIS   21
- PRINCIPLE EVALUATION ZONES   22

ABDOMINAL PALPATION   24

NECK PALPATION   28
- SCM ZONE   29
- TRAPEZIUS ZONE   31

BACK PALPATION   33

ACU-ZONE TREATMENT PART 1: ESSENTIAL TREATMENT   35
- YIN TANG – HALL OF IMPRESSION   36
- BL 2 – GATHERED BAMBOO   38
- TAI YANG – GREAT YANG   40
- DU 17 – BRAIN'S DOOR   42
- BL 9 – JADE PILLOW   44
- GB 12 – MASTOID PROCESS   46

ACU-ZONE TREATMENT PART 2: SUPPORT TREATMENT   49
- HUATUO JIAJI AT THE LEVEL OF L5 (HJL5)   50

Kd 1 – Bubbling Spring	52
GB 26 – Belt Channel	54
GB 25 – Essence Gate	56
Du 14 – Great Vertebra	58
SI 13 – Crooked Wall	60

ACU-ZONE TREATMENT PART 3: SYNTHESIS TREATMENT — 63

Lu 7 – Broken Sequence	64
LI 4 – Joining Valley	66
ST 43 – Sunken Valley/Outer ST 43	68
Sp 4 – Grandfather Grandson	70
Ht 5 – Penetrating the Interior	72
SI 3 – Back Stream	74
BL 62 – Extending Vessel	76
Kd 6 – Shining Sea	78
Pc 6 – Inner Gate	80
SJ 5 – Outer Gate	82
GB 41 – Foot Governor of Tears / GB 42 – Earth Five Meetings	84
Lr 3 – Great Rushing	86

IMPORTANCE OF THE BRAIN STEM: A WESTERN MEDICAL PERSPECTIVE — 88

WALK-THROUGH OF ACUPUNCTURE TREATMENT — 92

VITAL ENERGY MUSCLE (VEM) TESTING — 98

LOCATION OF TEST POINTS — 106

HERBAL PRESCRIPTION PROCESS — 108

HEAT THERAPY IN TREATMENT — 111

POST-ACUPUNCTURE TREATMENT FINE-TUNING AND CARE — 112

CASE STUDIES — 113

CONCLUSION — 135

BIBLIOGRAPHY — 137

BIOGRAPHY — 138

ACKNOWLEDGMENTS

I would first like to thank all my teachers, including Kiiko Matsumoto with whom I have learned for over 20 years. Thanks to her I was really able to develop this technique. I am also grateful for the teachings of the late Ryosuke Uryu, who inspired my own VEM technique.

From the bottom of my heart I thank Mateo Bernal for understanding my awkward English and for dedicating so much time and for his wonderful writing ability. Deep thanks to Seishiro Hokazono, who was instrumental in translating and editing.

Thanks also to David Myers, D.O. for his editing and suggestions.

A deep thanks to Rita Danis for her wonderful cover art.

Thanks to Sonia and Andrea for their support and help in my clinic, and for their work on the video.

Above all I am thankful for my patients, who are my best teachers, who have given me more than 80,000 treatment opportunities to learn.

And thank you to all those who have supported me on my path.

ON THIS REVISED EDITION

Since first publishing this book a year ago, I have encountered some better techniques and instructions.

- Please take a look at page 19 about additional Synergetic Qi technique. It is helpful for neck and deeper tissue tenderness. I found that a practitioner can guide qi to flow freely and deeply with just touching the target tenderness
- Adding Lu 7, Pc 6, SI 3 is helpful to alleviate soreness in SCM with more variant conditions
- Using Seirin # 03 (0.10x15mm) enables me treat small children and sensitive patients with ease
- Please check the description of each acupuncture point and zone for updates

Finally, I would like to thank David Myers D.O. for checking every page and word of my book for corrections, and Seishiro Hokazono LAc for translating my original Japanese thinking and writing to more easily understood English. Only with their help, could I publish this revision. I appreciate their dedication. Many thanks go to my family and clinic staff that supported me throughout the year.

August 24, 2014
Masaaki Nakano, DOM

HOW I HOPE YOU WILL BENEFIT FROM THIS BOOK

- This is a system which is simple and easy to learn, and will translate into immediate results in your clinical practice
- It is a comfortable system which employs gentle techniques, with which patients resonate easily
- You are encouraged to think deeply to arrive at elegant and refined acupuncture treatments; It is based on the selection of among 25 total points, using fewer than 10 needles per treatment
- This system offers an effective clinical strategy of acupuncture and herbal prescription which does not rely on tongue or pulse diagnosis
- It is ultimately a practical technique, intended to be very useful even in the busiest clinics
- Volume 1 gives you strategies to understand and treat pain

FOREWARD

I met Dr. Nakano one afternoon at a teashop in Las Cruces. I had moved to the small town to join a friend in his clinic. New Mexico required that I wait six months to take its board examination to be able to practice in the state, so in the meantime I was doing manual labor picking pecans and working as a receptionist at my friend's clinic in order to make ends meet. Needless to say, I was craving the intellectual and magical inspiration of Chinese medicine that I had come to love in school and in practice elsewhere. Someone came in to the clinic and mentioned in passing that they had gotten acupuncture from another guy in town who, "did a lot of pressing on my abdomen," at which point my eyes lit up and I thought to myself, "Maybe there is somebody else in town I can connect with about Japanese-style acupuncture." I was hoping to simply find somebody with whom I could share experiences and have collegial banter. I had no idea that I would find Dr. Masaaki Nakano, master acupuncturist, and open-hearted teacher.

I called Dr. Nakano's office and set up a meeting with him - I told him I was a new practitioner in town and wanted to get to know him. Graciously he accepted and found time to meet with me over the weekend for a tea.

Dr. Naka, as I would come to refer to him, sat with me on that first day for nearly four hours. Our free-flowing conversation was not so much about acupuncture theory or methods or techniques or special point protocols, but about our approach to medicine. This is how we first connected. Dr. Naka would talk to me about his ideas of healing and disease, about seeing the patient as a whole, about his own approach and his personal challenges. Immediately I recognized a deep sense of humility in Dr. Naka. It is one of his most endearing and respectable qualities. He shared honestly with me about his first years as a practitioner, not feeling confidence in himself and having mixed results with patients. He found no need to try to put himself on any pedestal, which made it very easy and natural for me to continue to listen and to be open to him, as I usually have very little tolerance for teachers with huge egos. But his honesty and sincerity were disarming for me, and compelling. He could relate to me and I to him in that sense. But it also told the story of how he began his search for what would become his method of acupuncture. His desire to help his patients, and listen openly to their feedback, was the impetus for exploring new techniques. It is natural that we, as practitioners, encounter difficulties when we treat our patients. Not all patients respond the same to acupuncture, not all patients with the same conditions respond the same. A question of major importance to us as practitioners is how we answer those challenges, those gaps in our knowledge or ability.

This book is based on hours of recorded and spontaneous conversations between Dr. Naka and I. While on the surface his technique seems simple, it is by no means easy. I have labored to elaborate on his philosophies and underlying concepts because it is my deep belief that they are of critical importance in his success. There is clearly more going on in his treatments than the simple and correct selection of points. When I observe him work I often see remarkable, almost magical, if not implausible, results. Seeing is believing, and I regularly saw these things in the clinic. It led me to question, "Why does this work?" and, "What is *really* going on here?" These questions that I asked were also the ones that led him to develop these techniques. Incessant questions, almost childlike, to understand and to be curious about acupuncture, are the source of this technique, and I believe that we can all benefit from this spirit, this approach, when learning this method. I had long heard that acupuncture is an art, but I had yet to see the true acupuncture artist. This concept had been, up to meeting him, a myth. One that I believed in, that inspired me, but was something that I had not experienced. It took all of five minutes in the clinic watching him work to realize that I was in the presence of an artist. The skill and fluidity, the completeness of his work, and the shear ability to take a step so far back as to truly be considered global, left me in awe. It also left me feeling like an infant, just being able to crawl while I watch someone dance. He is one who has the ability to deftly coordinate dozens of fine movements and theories with apparent effortlessness. I have experienced this with different martial arts masters, with those who are able to put theory of fluidity and receptivity into practice. When people see those masters in action they almost always say, "The way he *moves* is beautiful." They rarely comment on individual skills or techniques. It is the totality of their movement which separates them from the beginners - something that is almost beyond words, only really summarized by describing their "movement" because it is not just one piece, but the integration into a whole that is so striking.

I have been fortunate enough to spend hours and days with Dr. Naka, because he has been so generous with his time and knowledge, and seems to have endless energy and passion when discussing acupuncture and his methods. So eager to teach, and to share. I have heard him tell people that, "Acupuncture for him is like his endorphin rush - it makes me happy. Some people seek sky diving. I love coming to the clinic." Over these meetings with him our conversations would often shift to our personal lives and experiences. I learned how he first came to the US in order to ride his bicycle from Los Angeles to New York City because he dreamed of seeing the statue of liberty. Day after day, Dr. Naka seems curious, excited, and interested in his work. Never a dull moment, each person is so new. I hope that his approach, his example, his life - Masaaki Nakano as a whole person - inspires you as much as me.

Mateo Bernal

Las Cruces, NM 2013

PREFACE

"Time flies like an arrow"

I continued thinking about how to address the patient's pain, to ease his or her suffering somehow, and the days and months flowed for 23 years.

"When does my clinic become that to which many patients come? When can I get confidence with acupuncture treatment and prescribing Chinese medicine? How do I know when my treatment has helped?"

Finally since the days of the first year of my practice which were marked by my worry at these questions, many of the answers have been brought to light.

I opened a clinic, like you, after graduating school. I practiced the theory and techniques which were studied in school, and despite my best intentions to study hard and practice diligently, I witnessed only mixed results. This book is written thanks to years of frustration, fear, and insecurity. At the time, of course, I didn't see much benefit of such feelings. But they led me to search and dig for answers. The practitioner that has emerged from this crucible understands the importance of challenges and difficulties in order to open a new path.

Therefore, the Traditional Chinese Medicine (TCM) which we studied in school may appear considerably different than the method that I have developed. This is not a critique of TCM – far from it. This is meant to augment the body of knowledge of any person who practices Chinese medicine. If you have reached a plateau in your own practice, or don't feel satisfied with results you are getting in the clinic, then I can relate. In this we have a shared experience, and perhaps you will benefit from my process. I just ask that you keep an open mind and give this method an honest chance.

I graduated from a standard TCM program in the US. Like many students, I felt a bit like a baby bird pushed out of the nest – encouraged to fly but not sure if I yet could. After school I decided I needed more training to feel confident, so I travelled to China to apprentice in hospitals for months where I studied with different masters, covering theory, moxibustion, acupuncture, herbal medicine, Tuina, and even qigong. I returned to the US to begin practicing what I had learned and seen. The treatments I observed in China were very strong – typically large-gauge needles, deep insertion, and strong manipulation. This caused a lot of discomfort in the patients. However, in China it seemed that patients either didn't mind or they accepted that this was simply how it was. I also saw that the way Chinese medicine was practiced there was compartmentalized – acupuncture in one wing, Herbs in another, Tuina in another, and in some places, even Western medicine and labs were available.

In any educational program there are bound to be some contradictions. I learned, like all of us, that in theory Chinese medicine is a holistic one. In practice, however, I saw otherwise. And despite the rhetoric, I also didn't see too much concern with the experience of the patient. Huge over-crowded hospitals and over-worked doctors had to direct their attention to quantity rather than quality. Their treatment protocols were often geared at being able to accommodate the largest number of people per hour rather than focusing on the individual. This, and the separation of treatment modalities, discouraged integration and holistic, individualized treatments for the patient. People typically received protocols for their ailments. They were explained that treatment takes time, they should return every day or two or three times per week. It seemed that the pain that happened during the acupuncture treatment was normal, and that the patient should simply accept that this was a part of the process. I saw that this may work in China, but in the US, and in my native Japan, it was much different. In private clinics, where people paid for their acupuncture services, they demanded quick results and a pain-free experience. I found that if I caused pain to my patients at my clinic in the US they often didn't return, or complained later. The final straw came when a couple weeks after a treatment, I got a call from an attorney saying the patient he represents had a condition that had been aggravated from the treatment. Fortunately, we discovered that nothing was wrong with the treatment, and it simply required explaining to the patient to reassure them that all was well. Getting a call from a lawyer really shook me up, and I didn't want that to happen again. But these experiences led me to search for a safer, more relaxing, and demonstrably effective method of acupuncture. Since then I have not used local acupuncture nor electrical stimulation.

The treatments that I learned in school and in China were based on the idea that instant feedback from the patient was not necessary. The physician was supposed to be guided by the tongue and pulse - a positive change in pulse indicated the success of the treatment, and the patient would be notified that there was progress, and even if they experienced no change during the treatment, they should continue to come because the practitioner observed an improvement in their pulse. This was frustrating to both patients and to myself because people were often leaving his clinic with the feeling of, "I am not sure anything happened here today…" This was another reason for me to seek out a new method.

Palpation-based acupuncture, as popularized in the US by practitioners like Kiiko Matsumoto, was the answer that I was searching for. It provided immediate feedback to both the practitioner and to the patient, and the gentle yet powerful techniques caused no pain or ill side-effects.

At the end of the day, our job is to provide the best care we can to our patients. It is incumbent upon us to stay open and keep searching for better methods that will benefit our patients, constantly adapting and trying new things if necessary. With that in mind, I had to leave behind a lot of ideas that were at the core of my education. My current approach, which combines a gentle acupuncture technique, limited point selection, and the frequent combination of herbal formulas, is the culmination of 23 years of clinical experience. The time in the clinic has been my best guide, and patients have been my best teachers. By listening to them I have tried to learn what helps, what doesn't, and what is most comfortable and effective at the same time.

What I have developed is unique and, above all, practical. These methods are based on clinical practice and results, and supported by theory, not the other way around. Theory is truly important, and I am constantly referring to the classics. This guides and augments my clinical practice. At the end of the day what is truly important is your work and results in the clinic. If not, why else do we spend so much time studying? We are not here for simply philosophical entertainment, after all!

My search for a new method was in part based on the fact that my education was highly theoretical, and many times in the clinic things didn't play out like they did in the textbooks. Rarely did a person come in with a "textbook" case of a TCM pattern. They almost always presented with a complex pattern which was a combination of often conflicting conditions. What is the strategy in treatment? We learned how to address individual patterns, and were given herbal formulas and point combinations to deal with these, but what do you do when the person doesn't present like in the textbook? Any system should ultimately be practical. This is the reason why I felt compelled to share this system with others – I observed that after more than 20 years of clinical practice I finally found a demonstrably and utterly practical system which can be of benefit to many practitioners who are open to thinking a bit outside the box and to their patients who will doubtless appreciate the results.

One day, many years ago, I had the privilege of shadowing the great late Master Nagano in his clinic in Japan. I spent the day with him, and witnessed impossible results. "I want to be like this one day," I said to myself. I realize that I had set the bar high. But of all the conversations that we had, one stayed etched deeply in my mind. Master Nagano said that he had a limited capacity in this world – that his healing had to be limited to his clinic. But if he was able to share or teach his method, it was a way to extend his healing impact. This sentiment, at the heart of my practice, is what guides this book. I believe that healing is possible, and I hope that through this technique many others will be able to benefit from the wisdom passed down to me.

INTEGRATED SYNERGY THERAPEUTICS

It would be beneficial to begin with defining the name – *Integrated Synergy Therapeutics* - which is what I have decided to call this system, as well as the title of this book, Practical Oriental Medicine. In Volume 1 I have decided to focus on the fundamentals of the treatment of pain. Future volumes will address internal disorders, such as allergies and hormonal balance.

Synergism

Fundamentally, this system uses the concepts of zones to understand the physiology of the body. By understanding the body according to broad zones, we are able to integrate traditional Chinese theories such as meridians and organs with Western concepts such as nerve pathways, neurochemicals, and brain stem theory. This is the *Synergism*. In this system you will not find diagnoses, but rather an observation of the involvement of various zones. Zones can include energetic, traditional meridian-based and Zang-fu disorders combined with their physical manifestations along the various trajectories of the body. This system integrates the elegant and elaborate mapping of energetic and physical pathways described in terms such as primary meridians and divergent pathways as well as the quality of *qi* that flows within them, such as nutritive or protective *qi*. Modern science and medicine have given us the ability to observe the physical happenings in the body as never before in history. This system does not deny any modern understandings of physiology, but strives to understand it in the context of the very complete system we have been handed down over the millennia. Rather than strictly adhering to dogma or tradition, the wisdom of this system is the product of listening to our patients and trying to discover what will be of most benefit to them. In that way, the system is constantly shifting according to new information, and I hope that it never becomes static.

Synergetic Qi

In the context of this system the term is deliberately used instead of *qi*, which is a Chinese word and concept. A more full exploration of the notion of *Synergetic Qi* will come later. For now what is necessary to understand in order to appreciate the name of this system is that it is not only the physical body that we work with, but the energetic one as well. As acupuncturists, this is what we manipulate. As the ancient books say, move the *qi* and the physical will follow. This is at the heart of this system. A more complete understanding of *Synergetic Qi* is to realize that it is also consciousness – that of the patient as well as that of the practitioner. The power of the mind and positive thinking, intention, and focus are very important elements of this system. To me, *qi* comes from a connection between the patient and the practitioner – it is a combination. It is more than just an isolated *qi* that is manipulated in the patient's body with the acupuncture needle. Healing comes from the *synergy* of the practitioner's consciousness as well as the patient's *qi*.

Practical Oriental Medicine

Above all, this system is intended to be clinically practical to the reader. After years of struggling to reconcile theory and clinical practice, this is the system that has emerged. Bottom line – if it doesn't work in the clinic, it is not useful. We need to explore ways to make our treatments more and more effective, and this system strives to be eminently practical.

SIMILARITIES AND DIFFERENCES BETWEEN IST AND TCM

For the sake of clarity, perhaps it is useful to highlight some commonalities and divergences between TCM, which is the predominant system of Chinese medicine taught in the US, and Integrated Synergy Therapeutics.

There are far more similarities than differences, although it may help us understand some of the nuances of this system if we can attempt a comparison between the two systems.

First of all, Integrated Synergy Therapeutics is based on the same foundational principles as TCM. Both systems believe in the meridian systems that are the conduits and regulators of *qi* in the body. By manipulating different points along these trajectories, we are able to exert change across the entire system, and not simply in the local area where a needle is placed. In TCM, this would be called "point actions", suggesting that each point on the body has a number of actions that are effected when needled. Points are chosen based on diagnosis of either Zang-Fu, 8 Principles, Wen Bing or Shang Han Lun disease progression and treatment principles, etc. Herbal formulas are often added to enhance the efficacy of the acupuncture treatment.

Much the same can be said for IST. In IST, however, points are not chosen on their empirical or historical point actions and indications, but rather as representatives of zones which are most affected in the patient. The practitioner reaches the conclusions about which zones are affected by direct palpation of the body. After the zones are selected, appropriate points are chosen which have a broad regulating effect on the zone in order to open the zone, harmonize the imbalance within it, and integrate the zone back into the body and brain. In IST, local, tender, *ah-shi* points are never chosen for treatment.

TCM	IST
Local tender points (*ah shi*) often considered for treatment points.	Local points never chosen for treatment – only used for evaluation of improvement of condition and for zone selection.
Sensation of "*de qi*" is necessary response at site of needle insertion. Stimulation is required so that the patient "feels" the *qi*.	All sensation at point of insertion is discouraged – the patient should scarcely realize that the needle has been placed. *De qi* is not encouraged at all.
Point actions and indications are used to determine point selection based on diagnosis.	Palpation of neck, abdomen, back and areas where patients complain of pain determines point selection.
Diagnosis and differentiation of pattern based on tongue and pulse.	Palpation of neck, abdomen, back and areas where patients complain of pain determines diagnosis.
Pattern differentiation at the center of diagnosis.	Zones are diagnostically significant rather than pattern differentiation.
Efficacy of treatment determined by long-term improvement.	Immediate response by body indicates efficacy of treatment.
Based on intimate knowledge of internal, external, extraordinary, and secondary meridians	Based on intimate knowledge of internal, external, extraordinary, and secondary meridians.
Typical course of treatment includes making a diagnosis, and choosing the correct points and sticking with for a course of treatment. After a course of treatment, adjustments can be made to the diagnosis and point selection.	Each treatment requires re-evaluation of patient, and new points may be selected. If the same points are used it is because palpation and release of evaluation zones yielded the same points.
Point selection guided by theory and empirical knowledge of point energetics and actions.	Points in this book also have "indications" associated with them, but they should not be used in the traditional way of selecting a point based on its indication alone – palpation is the principle guide to point selection.
Herbal formulas based on zang-fu and pattern differentiation, as well as tongue and pulse.	Selection of herbal formulas based on zang-fu and pattern differentiation, as well as VEM testing.
In TCM school, most theories on the Eight Extraordinary Meridians taught come from Shi Si Jing Ta Hui (Essays on Acupuncture and Moxibustion by Hua Bo Ren, 1341).	IST draws primarily on Chinese and Japanese sources, such as Qi Jing Ba Mai Kao (Research on the Eight Extraordinary Channels by Li Shi Zhen, 1578) and Wakan-sansai-Zue (Detailed Encyclopedia of Japanese and Chinese Culture and Customs compiled by Ryoan Terashima, 1713).
Requires the four observations in order to guide treatment.	Requires spending a great deal of time with each patient using palpation in order to understand the terrain of their body so as to understand their pathology and be guided to their healing.

PRACTICAL ACU-ZONE THERAPY

This system combines three complimentary methods, which will be described below. These are known as the "Essential treatment", "Support treatment," and the "Synthesis treatment". By using this system, one is able to simultaneously address the primary cause, or root, as well as the condition for which the patient has requested help, also known as the branch.

First of all, let's explain the basic "rules":

1. Start from the center and move out – from Ren or Du Channels and then move out.
2. No matter what the disease may be, treatment is done by selection of ten or fewer points out of the 25 points used in this system.
3. The patient should never experience pain during needling.
    a. A significant caveat is that the patient may experience discomfort as you palpate the various evaluation zones and/or where they complain of pain. This is not unusual – but you must remind them that this is an important part of the process both to inform the body of the healing message as well as to give both of you a point of reference for improvement, this treatment and the subsequent. For accurate evaluation, we must carefully palpate, discover and mark the tender areas. Both the patient and the practitioner will see the results.
    b. Another important aspect is that you should encourage good communication with the patient, constantly checking in with them about what you are doing and asking how they are feeling.
4. Palpation is of equal importance to acupuncture in this system. Without relevant palpation, this method would be empty of meaning and be another collection of point actions and indications.
5. Point selection is primarily based on palpation, but informed and guided by theory. The indication that a point has been selected properly is the effective release of tenderness at evaluation areas verified by palpatory diagnosis. This is not theoretical point selection based on pulse or tongue diagnosis, it is based on immediate reduction of tenderness at the evaluation zones. Simply put: if the tenderness is not relieved, the point is not correct. Points in this book also have "indications" associated with them, but they should not be used in the traditional way of selecting a point based on its indication alone – palpation is the principle guide to point selection.
6. A hallmark of this style is immediate reduction in symptoms of pain at evaluation zones and/or the site of pain. This should happen during the treatment.
7. Multiple treatments may be necessary to address the patient's complaints.

8. Regardless of the patient's complaints, the release of the important evaluation zones must be achieved – this is critical for the success of the treatment. This system is based on the understanding that the body and mind operate as a whole, contiguous unit, and the goal of the treatment is to facilitate communication. Once communication has been properly established, healing will happen on its own. This is why it is not important to use local points and why we focus so much on release of the neck, back, and abdomen.
9. Try not to compartmentalize symptoms. Unity rather than division. There are no points for "headache" or for "insomnia" in this system. If points are selected for the symptom of headache, it is because they release the affected zone. Always try to map the complaints together with the palpation picture that is revealed to guide you to the appropriate zone. For example, a female patient may complain of headache at the frontal and temporal areas, and presents with neck tenderness at the right side of C3, has abdominal tenderness at Ren 12, under the right ribcage, and bilaterally at the ST 29 area. How can we choose one point that will address all of her complaints simultaneously? A TCM approach might include LI 4, LI 11, Lr 3, GB 20, and ST 36, needled bilaterally. Understanding the body in zones can help us narrow our selection. I would first select an "Essential Point", in this case, *Yin Tang*, in order to address the Ren Channel. After which, I re-palpate the abdomen and neck and check in with the patient about her headache. If symptoms still exist, I continue with the treatment. Very likely I would choose the right *Liver 3* point to address the neck and subcostal tenderness, which are indicative of *Liver Zone* involvement. My treatments are often as simple as this.
10. Always move from big to small – we always begin with palpation, followed by the Essential points, and gradually make minor adjustments at the end. The first part of the treatment is about getting the big picture of the patient, and as you work with them, their body will guide you to do the fine-tuning. You can think about this like looking for the source of the problem. Focus first on main symptoms or current or acute symptoms.
11. Focus on the main complaint of the patient. This is what we start to work with on the patient.

Our goal is patient satisfaction. This style of treatment requires much on the part of the practitioner:
1) Must be able to think quickly and adjust in real-time.
2) Must be able to carry theory and maps in your head to be constantly analyzing and influencing your treatment.
3) Must have patience in getting results.
4) Must trust the system – don't give up too soon! A common mistake for beginners is to lose confidence when their point selection doesn't immediately yield results. Keep trying – the system works, you may just need to fine tune things. Maybe your point

selection is slightly off. Maybe the needle needs more gentle vibrations. Maybe you chose an incorrect point!

Of course, since almost all the patients have chronic components to their chief complaint, it is unreasonable to expect a full recovery after one treatment.

We are not sure how long the amelioration will last – this is not our measure of progress. That we get results during the treatment is the key, and their prognosis depends greatly on many factors, including their general health, constitution, diet, and lifestyle. The key here is, however, that the improvement in their condition during the treatment is what indicates that we are on the right track with their healing process.

One advantage of this system is that we are able to treat multiple problems in various parts of the body at the same time with fewer than ten needles. Unlike other systems, we treat the person and their condition as a whole and do not separate their problems to be dealt with one by one. We focus on the patient's chief complaint, but at the same time we don't treat the patient piecemeal.

THEORY

Definition of a zone

Zones includes primary, divergent, sinew, internal and external channels, so we don't necessarily need to diagnose whether the imbalance is external or internal. Carpal tunnel is a good example – pain in the wrist may be due to an "internal" disorder.

Zones are a simple way to see connections between internal and external, and for us it is not necessary to diagnose which one.

What is disease? What is health?

There are several perspectives we can take to understand health, disease, and healing – all inform one another and should be used interchangeably. *Integrated Synergy Therapeutics* (IST) is a system which allows for fluidity and free-flow between concepts in Western medicine and Oriental medicine. We can take from both to give us a well-rounded and complete understanding. While the theories of Oriental medicine are in fact able to explain health and disease, why not use the detailed anatomical, visual, and medical information available to us through science and imaging? These systems are not mutually exclusive. In fact, they inform one another. I have heard it explained as such: The two medicines are like the right and left eyes: when used at the same time they provide depth and perspective; alone we are left with a one-dimensional image. I strive to understand clinical practice through any theories or models available. Sometimes it is more convenient to choose a meridian-based explanation to understand palpation or point selection, other times I may choose dermatomes.

At the foundation of my practice is the belief that there is an existing healing network in the body, each organ functions to try to get the information to other organs. In the simplest of terms, when communication happens between organs, tissues, and the brain, there is health. The body is entirely capable of auto-regulation of fantastically complicated body rhythms such as cardiac rate and breathing as well as hormonal and endocrine functions, and so on. Due to trauma, stress, toxic exposure, physical strain or climactic factors, the body can get out of balance. This can happen gradually and in small increments or acutely and massively. This imbalance is a problem of communication in the body. The role of the acupuncturist is to help restore healthy communication throughout the body and its innate healing ability will take over. I often tell my patients, "I never cure you. The body cures itself." I believe that if I can help the body get back on track, it will take over and do what it naturally does best. I am aware that "life happens," and my role is to gently remind the body of what it already knows how to do.

This philosophy implies that both "internal" disorders, such as organ dysfunction and chemical imbalance, as well as "external" disorders, such as pain and musculoskeletal issues, are both treated with the same approach: encourage and re-establish lines of healthy communication and trust that the body will heal itself.

If the nervous system isn't transmitting the right information, organs will not function at their healthy capacity. This is when disease occurs.

The brain is the center, and messages go from there to all organs, tissue, bones, etc. If there is damage or pain in the finger, the information should go to the brain and then be transmitted to the appropriate tissue or organ for a response. Disease or pain is a result of poor or incorrect information or poor transmission of information. In Oriental medicine, we call this *qi* blockage or stagnation. If there is a blockage somewhere, *qi*, Blood or Body Fluids (for me this is synonymous with lymph) isn't flowing or communicating information correctly.

From this perspective, all that is necessary is macro-regulation, broad integration, and communication. This is why so few points are used in the system. This is also why the "essential" points of this system are located on the head. And given the predominant theories about Extraordinary channels and their function in broad regulation of *qi* in the body, we can easily see why so many of the master points are integrated into this system.

One reason we palpate is to find where there is blockage, which typically manifests as tender spots. Usually there are multiple problems – not just one channel or area. It is usually multiple pathways of channels or along dermatomes. This is why I don't start with meridians, but I start with the brain - which is the center of it all. I get healing messages flowing through the meridians or nervous system.

This is why I palpate the neck, back, or abdomen. These are commonly where the biggest areas of blockage can show up.

The system is based on the idea of reestablishing communication. The neck is a bridge between heaven (the head) and earth (the body). In western medicine the neck, especially the upper cervicals, has a strong influence on the brain, and the brachial plexus on blood and oxygen to the arms. The neck is a very complex area with a lot of crossing points and many channels passing through. C3 seems to be critically important in this diagnostic system. By relieving pain at the Huatuo Jiaji points of either side of this vertebrae, the rest of the neck and shoulders typically release and the prognosis of the patient is much better.

Acupuncture and Channel Theory

We are looking at the body as a whole, a complete healing network system, not just a collection of individual problems. This is why we try to find points and how they overlap and layer rather than using individual points for individual pain and coming up with an incoherent or piecemeal treatment approach. Ideally, if you are palpating correctly and helping you and the patient find connections in the body, only a few points are necessary. And you are left with a very simple, elegant, and above all easy to understand and coherent message.

We know that each point on the channel is capable of doing many things through its various connections throughout the body. Something that was difficult for me in school was that a point was considered to typically have one indication but when it worked for other things we would stretch the theory to make it fit. We could say, "Wow, *Liver 3* helped with headache this time, why?" And we would look at the internal pathway of the Liver channel or the tendino-muscular channel. We know that opening the healing along a channel can have broad systemic effects, this is the basis of our medicine and a foundation of the channel theory – that all things are interconnected. However, it is incumbent upon us to figure out how to provide a coherent message that the body will understand based on our knowledge of the internal pathways of the body as well as faith that when we activate the *qi* it will go where it needs. We can come up with elaborate ways of explaining almost all therapeutic interactions through the channels or the five elements. This is not a critique of the models of the five element or channels, because they are fantastic metaphors for explaining all the infinitely interconnecting relationships in the body. What we need to do is figure out what is consistently practical that works for us in the clinic.

The fact that everything is connected is virtually undeniable, western and eastern medicines are converging on this concept. But this does not help us with therapy. It does not mean we can just put a point anywhere on the body and it will be helpful. IST offers a systematic approach to understanding the connections in the body and using them practically in the clinic. A simple, natural message is integrated in the body very easily. The goal of our treatment process is to provide a simple healing message to the body by establishing networks and communication and then let the broad healing happen and the internal functions to regulate themselves.

Concept of Synergetic Qi

Synergetic Qi is a very important concept in the practice of acupuncture and Oriental medicine. Qi is often defined simply as "energy" but it is much more than that. It has to do with exchange and communication. It has to do with interaction; Qi builds when there is interaction. It is also about vibration of energy. In Japanese this is called *Hado* – in English perhaps the best term is *resonance*. It is about how things resonate, or vibrate, with each other. Treatment is helping bring the body back into balance, helping yin and yang communicate in a conscious way.

Messages have to be sent in a conscious way. Verbal issues are important – many times I hear a patient say, "Stupid elbow!" I rarely hear people say, "Thank you for letting me know that the problem is here so I can help it. " These negative vibrations are powerful for the area.

From the therapist's side, you must stay positive, and there must be the right state of mind - "I can help." Many people start thinking, "What are the right points to use?" or, "What is the right diagnosis?" They focus on their own knowledge or techniques, but the more basic thing is wanting to help, having the right state of mind, and actually listening to the patient to see what their actual complaint is. Before starting to think about theory or treatment, connection with the patient must happen verbally or consciously. This is an important step, otherwise it is difficult to even begin therapeutic connection and interaction.

From the patient's side, the intention must be, "I want to feel better. I want to heal." Many have already given up or are very negative and defeated. The mindset must change. Eating, breathing, movement, consciousness/thinking, environment – 5 factors which are very important for healing. If one of these things feels unnatural for the body, it will tell you that you need to change or improve and we need to listen. This is why we get symptoms – they help guide us to what is out of balance.

You can learn technique and knowledge from this book, but understanding and cultivating the *qi* is very important and can take your practice to the next level. The therapist side of *qi* and patient side of *qi* are different and both must be considered. *Qi* flows in the direction from higher concentration to low concentration, so it is important for our *qi* to be healthy so that it may flow in the right direction and we are not taking from our patients. They will never get better this way! During the treatment, the intention of the practitioner is important. When I hold the needle and gently vibrate it, I am not letting my mind get distracted with anything else other than the treatment. I am constantly using my eyes and intention to guide the treatment from the needle to the target area for healing. For example, I insert the needle at Sp 4 and begin the gentle vibrations. After a moment I let my eyes drift to the left side of the abdomen, ribcage, and neck where there was tenderness upon palpation, all the while I continue the gentle vibrations. This allows for a special sort of "connection" to happen, between the needle, my eyes (and consciousness) and the healing target. This is another aspect of Synergetic Qi.

Synergy, as in the name of this system, means we combine knowledge, technique, and *qi* to get better therapeutic results with treatment.

Tools/Acupuncture Technique

I would like to introduce the tools that I use in my practice:

- NEEDLES – SEIRIN & TEMPO BRAND & PYONEX SINGLES (PRESS NEEDLE)
- FAR INFRARED FOOT SAUNA & TDP LAMP
- MOXSAFE SMOKELESS MOXA & SEIUN SMOKELESS INCENSE
- NON-TOXIC HIGHLIGHTER

Needle Stimulation

Needling happens to a shallow depth, by looking for the tight spot where the needle will immediately grab. The needle handle is grasped firmly with the fingers and gently vibrated until the tissue releases or relaxes. If you can't tell if the tissue is relaxing, just try for 10-20 seconds. Re-check the palpation zone. If pain remains, return and re-stimulate. If you still have pain after second stimulation, check point location. If after checking point location and still no release of area, you may need to choose another point.

When needling deeper points, like HJL5 or GB 25 and 26, I insert the needle slowly to a tight spot, or where it feels that the needle is "grabbed." This may involve changing the angle of the needle slightly until you find it. The patient should feel no pain. I gently vibrate the needle until the tension at the end of the needle dissolves.

Direction
Needles are always inserted in the direction of the flow of the channel

Technique/Qi of practitioner
Qi flows from high to low, so the acupuncturist must be healthy, and have an elevated level of *qi*. A very important technique crucial to making this treatment work has to do with making connections. It is important to look at the area you are focusing on while you are gently vibrating the needle. This allows for a subtle but important connection to be made in the patient's body between the treatment point and the healing target.

Additional Skill: Connection Technique
Once right points are needled with application of Synergetic Qi and more than 70% of tenderness is alleviated, you may want to release it further at deeper level. For an example of tenderness at Ren 12: You may hold a needle at Yin Tang with one hand (thumb and another finger) and hold Ren 12 with pads of 2nd and 3rd fingers of another hand. Apply 10~20 seconds of Synergetic Qi at Yin Tang while holding Ren 12 lightly. This should release the tenderness at Ren 12 further and at deeper level. This is applicable to other tenderness areas as well.

DIAGNOSIS

I was taught that diagnosis means that first you must diagnose, then you treat. Without a diagnosis, it is impossible to treat. For me it is a bit different, diagnosis and treatment happen simultaneously. Naming the diagnosis is not so important. In this system, a diagnosis might look more like "SCM tension" or "QL muscle/SI joint pain" based on discoveries from palpation, rather than a typical TCM diagnosis of Spleen *qi* deficiency or Liver *qi* stagnation or Kidney deficiency. Diagnosis is simply a statement of fact based on the condition of the body in real-time, today. This can also give us perspective on progress over time.

Treatment will depend on finding points that release the tension or pain at the diagnostically significant areas. There is not necessarily a one-to-one correlation between diagnostic zones and treatment points – the selection of points can vary depending on the global presentation of the patient in terms of their chief complaints, painful areas, diagnostically significant areas, and answers to general health questions such as digestion, sleep, etc. These questions which come from TCM can inform our treatment strategy by "lasering in" on a specific organ or channel disturbance. The relationships of organ, tissue, season, emotion, etc. that have been established in TCM are still valid and useful in this system, just maybe not of primary importance.

I am very concerned with diagnosis – no treatment can happen without it. In my practice I primarily use palpation of the body at various zones in order to arrive at treatment plans. Some people have been taught to use pulse and tongue diagnosis, and they are encouraged to continue to do so in their own practice to gather as much information as they can about the patient. However, based on years of clinical experience, I have found that abdominal, back, and neck palpation are more reliable and clear diagnostic measurements and I rarely examine the tongue or pulse.

PALPATORY DIAGNOSIS

Palpation is the beginning of treatment. It begins connections with the nervous system and channels to reintegrate and communicate. Relevant palpation is what we call the palpation of three areas:

1) areas that are of chief complaint to the patient, along with

2) adjacent areas and up/down associated channels

3) palpation of the principle evaluation zones of neck/abdomen/back

These three in combination comprise "relevant palpation." We could, theoretically, find painful or tender places all over the body. It is our job to figure out which areas are significant and useful in terms of treatment. Remember, this system is based on trying to connect the brain with the complex pattern of pain or disease that a patient presents with. This does not just happen with acupuncture – it begins with palpation. Our job is to figure out how to make sense of the patterns that the patient presents with and be able to distill an acupuncture treatment from that.

A case in point: Hegu, LI 4, one of the most commonly used points in Chinese medicine. We know that LI 4 may be used for Wind-Cold invasion, to promote sweating, for any problem of the head including headache, toothache, eye pain, stuffy nose, sinus problems, sore throat, as well as for low back pain, menstrual problems, general *qi* or Blood stagnation in the body manifesting as pain or tension anywhere in the body. The list goes on.

Depending on the school and teacher, we learn that there are so many possibilities for actions and indications of each point. How does the body know what to do with the information that we send it with the acupuncture needle? Palpation is how we refine the treatment, and simplify the message, so as to not confuse the brain.

Method of Palpation:

There are three levels of palpation, from shallow to deep. Palpation is done with the fingertips. You can use pads of the middle three fingers of either hand to palpate the abdomen, rather than using the whole hand. You can palpate in multiple directions in order to find the point. You are looking for tenderness at the reflex areas, and then mark the surface with a highlighter. It is common to use one color non-toxic highlighter, yellow for example, to mark the painful areas before treatment begins, and use a different color to mark points that remain after the different phases of the treatment as I go. This is done to be able to be sure of the efficacy of your treatment and correct point location or appropriate needle stimulation.

PRINCIPLE EVALUATION ZONES

Neck, Abdomen, Back

Reflex points or areas within these Evaluation Zones are what guide the treatment and give us the global picture. These Principle Evaluation Zones are the areas that are palpated on every patient, regardless of their complaint. First it must be determined whether the patient should be in prone, supine, or lateral recumbent position. Once you decide this, a supine patient will always have their neck and abdomen palpated along with wherever else is of chief concern to them. For the patient in the prone and lateral recumbent position, cervical, thoracic, and lumbar spines as well as their corresponding Huatuo Jiaji points are evaluated in addition to any other areas that the patient complains of pain or discomfort.

Phases:

Palpation is done in three phases. The first, and the most broad, is what will lead us to the selection of the Essential point or points. The next step is selecting the most powerful point to address the majority of the points remaining tender by using the Support or Synthesis points. The last point, if necessary, is the minute final adjustment to the treatment.

We begin with the Essential points, which go to the brain and therefore start at the most broad, non-specific level – yin or yang? We must palpate the front, back, or side of the body. This is how we arrive at the selection of Essential points.

After using the Essential points, we re-palpate and search for any remaining tender areas. Pain happens in layers - the brain primarily recognizes the worst pain. If there is anything left over, you have two options – Support treatment or Synthesis treatment points. We will choose points that cover the largest areas where any pain remains and keep working until we achieve no tenderness. This should be done with the fewest needles possible.

Palpation of Feet:

Palpation of the feet for temperature is very important in my clinical experience. I have noticed a strong correlation between cold feet and Yang deficiency, poor circulation, autonomic nervous system imbalance, and endocrine system especially thyroid and adrenal glands. Watching the changes in foot temperature of a patient over time is a helpful measure of the progress and prognosis of the patient. Sometimes people are not sensitive to their own cold feet, especially those who experience other heat signs, a good example being menopause, hot flashes and heat in the head, but careful examination of the feet will show coldness. One way to get around this is by using a simple non-contact thermometer to check the difference between temperature of head and feet. In most cases, you will see a significant difference, and it will help the patient become more aware.

Important!

The *order of palpation* is important: palpation should happen from the *center outwards*.

In other words, palpation always starts along the midline, whether that be the Ren or Du channels, and moves outward from there.

It is important to remember that we are working with zones – even if the patient has a chief complaint at the right shoulder, we must still palpate along the Du channel first when exploring the area. If the majority of tenderness in the area is along the Du channel, our first Essential point will be Du 17 rather than BL 9 or GB 12, which is indicated in right shoulder problems. It doesn't mean that we won't eventually use BL 9 or GB 12 on the right for that shoulder pain – we may – but it just means that we need to start with Du 17.

Another example: people may complain of pain all over the body, along the midline, both sides of the body, knees, shoulders, hands joints, etc. Where do we begin? Always start with the center line (whether that be on the front or back) and needle the appropriate Essential points, and then recheck the tender areas of the body and see what parts are left. In this way you will slowly be narrowing in on the details of the treatment. Remember: start from big and move to small.

We want to avoid using too many needles and strive for the simplest message possible. By starting along the midlines, we can eliminate a lot of "background noise" in the patient, and focus on what the patient's body really needs today.

ABDOMINAL PALPATION

Abdominal palpation is an important element of this system. I am not the first person to have abdominal palpation inform my treatments – there are countless practitioners and styles of acupuncture based on abdominal palpation theory and diagnosis. This is not intended to be an explanation of abdominal palpation, there are numerous books that are fantastic guides to the principles and theories of abdominal palpation. Here we will presume basic knowledge of abdominal palpation and discuss the nuances that this system offers.

Congruent with the rest of this approach, palpation of the abdomen is considered in zones. Zones may include front-*Mu* points but also often overlap with actual internal organ location and meridian pathways, both internal and external. Rarely are specific points palpated, but rather areas are considered to be significant; although individual and very specific points may be found to be tender, they may or may not correspond directly to traditional point locations along channels.

As stated previously, diagnosis and treatment are synonymous in this style. Therefore palpation of the zones merely guides us to treatment points. If the points work for the release of tenderness at the affected evaluation zone, then we have chosen the point correctly. But it would be false to understand these areas as "diagnostic zones" in the traditional sense of the word diagnosis. We do not draw diagnostic conclusions from information gathered during evaluation of these zones, and we certainly cannot infer disorder of internal organs from a Western perspective, for which laboratory testing is necessary.

We are given mere suggestions from the body as to where to begin our work – acupuncture treatment. The treatment points suggested for "clearing" these zones are what I have found, clinically and over time, to be commonly relevant and effective. But we cannot draw conclusions based on just one source of information. This system strives to integrate information, so we must find several sources of diagnostic information for us to be able to correctly select a point and, importantly, keep our point selection to a minimum. Put another way, if tenderness is found at the Lung Zone, we cannot simply conclude that Lu 7 is indicated. We must have several reasons to choose Lu 7:

1.) Is the point relevant to the patient's complaints and symptoms?
2.) Does the point release the tenderness at the Lung Zone?
3.) Does Lu 7 also address other tender evaluation areas, such as elsewhere on the abdomen or neck or back, especially Ren channel?

If you answered yes to all of these questions, then perhaps Lu 7 is the appropriate point. If not, keep searching. It may be another point that is more inclusive. Consider the global picture of the patient. For example, a patient may present with shortness of breath and digestive issues and the Lung Zone is tender. Perhaps the Spleen point is needled and reduces tenderness at the Spleen and Lung Zones (via Tai Yin connection). In this case Lu 7 is not needed at all. Another example: A patient presents with shortness of breath and perhaps a slight cough but also shows Kidney deficiency signs. Perhaps Kd 6 is what releases the Lung Zone as well as tenderness at the Kidney Zone. In this case, too, we can see how the overall presentation of the patient is important.

This kind of thinking applies to all point selection and your discernment includes distilling information gathered from neck, back, and abdominal palpation as well as relevant local palpation of areas of pain and other internal symptoms that the patient shares.

ZONES ON THE ABDOMEN

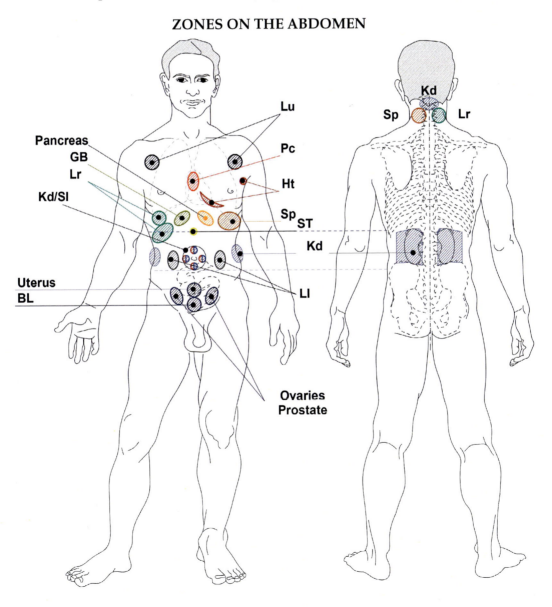

- Lung Zone: Lung 1 - 2 area
    - Essential Point first – could be BL 2
        - Then choose Lu 7 ipsilateral to Lung Zone tenderness
- Heart Zone: Sp 20, along sternum at Kd 22-25, ST 18 on left.
    - If Heart zone alone, without Pericardium Zone, BL 2 is first choice as essential point
        - Then Ht 5
- Pericardium Zone: More commonly used than Heart Zone - Ren 12 – 17
    - Yin Tang
    - (left) Pc 6
        - Left Sp 4 as a support point if Pc 6 doesn't fully release
- Liver Zone: Along and under right ribcage, in the anatomical area of liver. From sternum to corner of ribcage is GB area. From corner to tip of 11th rib is Liver zone (Lr 14 and GB 24 are Liver Zone)
    - The GB zone may indicate in internal Gall Bladder problem, but more likely during treatment it will be Liver point
        - Right BL 2
            - Then Lr 3 (right)
                - If still doesn't release, use (right) Pc 6 as support point
                - If the GB zone is the only area left, use right GB 41/GB 42
- Spleen and Pancreas – Left ribcage
    - From sternum to tip of the ribcage is Pancreas, from tip to 11th rib is Spleen area
        - Both are typically treated with the Spleen points
        - First left BL 2
            - Left Sp 4 as follow up
                - Support point is left Pc 6 or ST 43
- Stomach Zone: Between Ren 10 – 14
        - Yin Tang is first choice
            - Left side Pc 6
                - Support with left Sp 4
- Navel zone: Kd 16, Ren channel above and below navel Ren 7-9

*Choice of points is based on chief complaints and/or acupressure trials on different points

    - First point is Yin Tang
        - If Kidney signs or symptoms (low energy, cold feet, frequent urination, etc.)
            - Kd 6
        - If GI symptoms – Digestive issues, diarrhea/constipation, gas, bloating, etc.
            - SI 3
- Large Intestine Zone – bilateral ST 25 to ST 28 and Sp 13-15 area
    - Right side Lr 3, left side Sp 4
    - Could be LI 4 or ST 43
        - BL 2 is point of choice, depending on side where pain presents
            - Lr 3 or Sp 4 depending on other abdominal findings
        - Most important point is ST 43, support point is LI 4

- - - If one spot maybe use LI 4, but multiple spots left over could be more ST43. Remember, Sp 4 or Lr3 is the best, very powerful, and should release a lot of the pressure
- Kidney Zone: Tip of 12th rib (GB 25) and QL muscles (the area between BL 22-24 and 51-52)
  - Essential point: BL 2 if supine, (BL 9 if prone)
    - Kd 6 follows if BL 2 doesn't release
      - If tender at BL 23 area as well as GB 25-26 (Dai Mai) area
        - Use GB 41 as support point
      - If there are no internal signs that the Kidney is involved (i.e. adrenal fatigue, Kidney yin/yang deficiency signs), and the chief complaint seems more related to more external, musculo-skeletal issues
        - Support point can be BL 62
    - If you are unsure, you may use acupressure on both Kd 6 and BL 62 to determine which point releases the tenderness in the low back best.
- Bladder Zone: Ren 2-3
  - Essential point – Yin Tang
    - Follow-up point is Kd 6, check left and right and choose based on tenderness or release of Bladder Zone with palpation
    - Support point Lu 7, check left and right and choose based on tenderness or release of Bladder Zone with palpation
- Uterus Zone: Ren 3-4, Kd 12-13 area
  - Essential Point – Yin Tang
    - Support point Lr 3, check left and right and choose based on tenderness or release of Uterus Zone with palpation
    - If tenderness mostly along Kidney channel
      - Kd 6, check left and right and choose based on tenderness or release of Uterus Zone with palpation
- Lower Jiao Zone: Ren 4-6
  - This zone is not very specific by itself – it could indicate a disorder in the Lower Jiao generally, meaning San Jiao, Kidney, Large Intestine, Small Intestine (i.e. digestion) or Uterus, etc. Palpation of surrounding area should give you more information about how to interpret tenderness at this area.
    - Yin Tang is Essential Point
      - Support point is SI3
- Male – Prostate/Female – Ovaries: Kd 11-12/ST 29-30
  - Essential point is BL 2
    - Either Kd 6 or Sp 4 depending on where tenderness is

Important!
This palpation system is just a rough guide to help you narrow down your point selection. The key to point selection is to check with other symptoms and chief complaint, as each point can potentially cover multiple palpation zones.

NECK PALPATION

Palpation of the neck is a unique and critically important feature of this system. Palpation of the neck is often both the most consistently accurate and diagnostically relevant area of the body. In my experience, many people who come to the clinic, for one reason or another, don't present with any findings on the abdomen, making treatment difficult. Sometimes a very tense and strong man will come to the clinic, and despite having obvious tightness all over the abdomen, doesn't convey to the practitioner that he experiences any tenderness at those areas. In this case it is very difficult to try to make point selection. Another example is the person who comes to the clinic with a host of problems yet the abdomen reveals nothing in terms of tenderness or pain. In both cases, and in almost every patient, I have found that palpation of the neck almost always shows clear signs, easy for both the patient and myself to recognize.

Above all, it is a pragmatic approach to palpatory diagnosis. Additionally, it has other benefits. Internal organ imbalances will show on the neck, not just the abdomen. This is particularly true of digestive disorders. I have countless examples of chronic neck pain being alleviated by the treatment of the digestive system (Spleen/Stomach).

Autonomic nervous system imbalances will show in the neck as well. Stress, mental, and emotional tension, along with accompanying internal organ imbalances, can express as tenderness along the evaluation zones of the neck.

Lastly, structural issues, either local or distal, such as muscular inflammation, subluxation, and misalignment will show on the neck.

Palpation of the neck is essentially done over two zones: **SCM Zone** and **Trapezius Zone.**

SCM Zone

The sternocleidomastoid (SCM) muscle has 4 zones from top to bottom. These are found by dividing the SCM into four sections from the mastoid process to the two points of insertion on the sternum and clavicle.

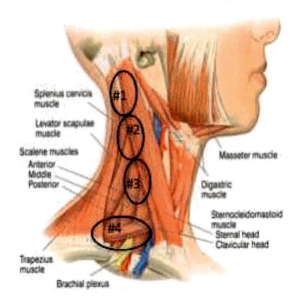

Palpation method:

The primary area is palpated behind the SCM (when patient is lying supine, you can grasp the SCM with your fingertips and the posterior border of the SCM is the line you will palpate along). The first of the three divisions of the SCM muscle is the most superior, close to the mastoid process. It is about two *cun* in length. The next two divisions are also about 2 *cun* in length each. This is an approximation. Use the pads of middle three fingers to palpate the whole width of SCM. Remember, we are considering zones here, not specific points. We have named the four divisions as SCM #1, SCM #2, SCM #3 and SCM #4 to help describe the significance of each zone and associated treatment.

- **SCM #1 –Atlas Reflex & SCM #2 –Lymph Reflex** (area slightly posterior to the SCM)
    - Primary treatment choice: Tai Yang
        - if face up – SJ 5
        - if face down – SJ 5
        - if side-lying – Supported by SJ 5
        - if Lung symptoms – Lu 7
- **SCM #3 –Subclavian Artery Reflex:** (area slightly posterior to the SCM)
    - Primary treatment choice: Tai Yang
        - if face up – SJ 5
        - if face down – GB 12
        - if side-lying - Supported by GB 12
        - if Heart symptoms – Pc 6

- **SCM #4** (Brachial Plexus Reflex – anterior and middle scalenes) – often found with accompanying tenderness at the other SCM divisions.
    - Tenderness at the Brachial Plexus Zone often shows with pain or tingling/numbness in the arm and hand, including carpal tunnel syndrome.

- Primary point: Tai Yang
  - This point should be palpated with the patient either face up or side-lying.
    - Secondary points: LI 4, ST 43
    - Remaining pain at posterior scalenes: SI 3

Treatment Strategy:

Any elimination of tension or pain at the SCM must fit in with the other findings on the neck, abdomen, and/or patient's chief complaints. This section is about general points to consider, but the SCM is not in a vacuum, and should not be treated this way in your acupuncture treatment. While we consider the release of tension along the SCM to be of critical importance to the health and prognosis of the patient, we must select points that consider the overall presentation of the patient.

In general, Tai Yang or SJ 5 should release SCM #1, 2, and/or 3. If any left over at #4, then choose brachial plexus point. If there is any lingering pain after needling Tai Yang, then you may choose a support point. Be sure that you are getting the appropriate release of tension at the SCM before you decide to move on to a support point. If after needling Tai Yang or SJ 5 you still have significant tenderness left over at #1,2, and/or 3, then it is likely that you need to adjust your point location or use 10-20 seconds more of gentle vibrations at the needle before seeking a support point. If after more vibrations at the needle and/or checking point location, you still have tenderness somewhere along the SCM, you should consider other complaints the patient may have, such as back pain, shoulder pain, or internal conditions. These will help you select a support point.

Remember: The support point won't do its job if the primary point is not selected correctly or the location is off.

Since we consider the findings at the SCM in relation to the rest of the body, below are examples of concurrent symptoms and treatment strategies when choosing support points.

- If the main symptoms of the patient are anywhere from their shoulder to their hand or even fingers, the point selected is usually GB 12. This point is palpated all around the mastoid process to determine the most tender area and needled precisely there.
- If there is Brachial Plexus Zone (SCM #4) tenderness but the patient presents with no symptoms of pain between the shoulder and hand, we may still consider LI 4 or ST 43. In order to choose which of these, we must factor in the internal disorders and symptoms that connect us to those points.
- If the patient presents with abdominal tenderness at the Stomach or Pericardium abdominal zones, then Pc 6 may be the appropriate point choice for releasing the SCM.

Trapezius Zone

Like the SCM Zone, the Trapezius Zone consists of four divisions, spanning from the occiput (BL 10 area) down along the Huatuo Jiaji points of the cervical vertebrae and across the middle fibers of the trapezius muscle to the GB 21 area.

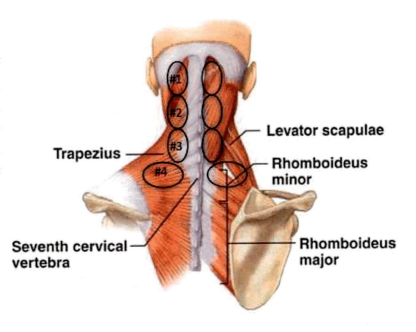

Palpation Method:

When patient is lying supine, you can gently grasp both sides of the neck and feel for the spine. With hands on either side of the spine, use index and middle fingers to check the Huatuo Jiaji points from the occiput down to C7, carefully checking and making observations about your findings at each of the four divisions. (On larger patients, you can use index, middle and ring fingers for palpation.)

TRAPEZIUS ZONES:

- **Trapezius #1:** (C1-C2) – upper fibers of Trapezius muscle and suboccipital muscle group)
    - If pain persists, think about Kidney involvement
        - Supine treatment: BL 2
            - Support point: Kd 6
        - Prone treatment: BL 9
            - Support point: BL 62
- **Trapezius #2** – C3-C4 **most important** Lr/Sp – upper fibers of Trapezius and splenius capitus and splenius cervicis muscles (which insert and attach at C1-C3 and T3-T6)
    - Left side tenderness – Spleen involvement
        - Treatment point is usually left Sp 4
    - Right side tenderness – Liver involvement
        - Treatment point is usually right Lr 3
- **Trapezius #3** – C5-C6 – upper fibers of trapezius
    - Treatment point should be SI 3

- **Trapezius #4** – middle fibers of the Trapezius muscles (GB 21, SJ 15) and levator scapula (which originates and inserts at C1-4 and superior angle and adjacent medial border of the scapula.)
  - Treatment points are usually SJ 5 or GB 12

Treatment Strategy:

There are basically two ways to release this zone, and these depend on what your other findings are on the abdomen as well as the patient's chief complaints.

First choice:

- Yin Tang - if abdominal palpation shows Yin Tang zone (Ren 2 – 15) *or*
- BL 2 – if there are no signs on the abdomen, or if Yin Tang zone is not tender

Second choice:
- If #1 Zone remains tender
  - Kd 6
- If #2 Zone remains tender
  - Lr 3 (right side) and Sp 4 (left side)
- If #3 Zone remains tender
  - SI 3
- If #4 Zone remains tender
  - If GB 21
    - Select GB 12 if other symptoms are only in the upper part of the body
    - Select GB 41 if other symptoms show in the lower part of the body
  - If SJ 15
    - Select SJ 5

BACK PALPATION

Palpation of the back consists of the spine, Huatuo Jiaji points, and BL channel. If a patient has a specific complaint on the back we also check the adjacent areas to where they complain of pain, and this can help lead us to more effective point selection.

Pain found in the Back Areas may be indicative of internal disorders (i.e. organ imbalances), or "external" disorders, such as muscular tension or structural imbalance, or both. Diagnostically, the areas on the back coincide very closely with the Back-Shu points and their associated organs.

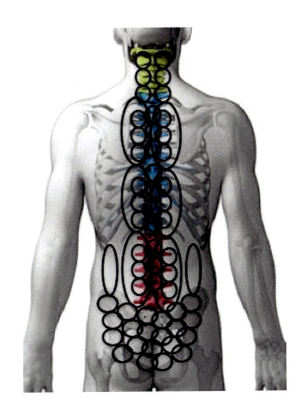

- *Upper Jiao Area*: Du 9 – 14 and BL 41 – 49 and the corresponding Huatuo Jiaji points (from C7-T7) for rhomboid muscles problems
    - This means that if there is a problem in the rhomboid muscles it may due to an internal organ condition (could be Lung, Pericardium, or Heart) or emotional stress, so we check those areas.
- *Middle Jiao Area:* T7-T12 (Du 6-9) and Jiaji points and BL 49 -46
    - Right side is Liver/Gallbladder reflection zone
    - Left side Spleen/Pancreas/Stomach zone
- *Lower Jiao Area:* L1-L5 (Du 3-Du 6) and Jiaji and BL 49 or 50 to Lumbar Eye point
    - Kidney reflection zone
- *SI Joint Area* (around S1 - S4 area and gluteus maximus origin)
    - Reflection zone for LI, SI, BL, uterus/ovaries, prostate
    - Palpate along the muscle fibers of the gluteus maximus where it originates at the sacrum and posterior iliac crest

Palpation Method:

Patient is palpated while lying prone or in lateral recumbent position on the table. Each intervertebral space from the occiput all the way to the sacrum is checked and marked if tender. As you are palpating the Du channel, you may also check the Huatuo Jiaji points as well.

Palpation of the spine is followed by palpation of the Bladder channel, both the inner and outer lines, and tender spots are carefully marked with the highlighter.

Treatment Strategy

Part of the palpation of the back includes marking all tender points that you find. After marking all points that you find to be tender, it may be challenging to come up with a clear treatment. As with the rest of this system, points are selected for multiple reasons with the goal of using the fewest possible points. This is only achievable if you choose points that will have the broadest-reaching influence and can cover multiple zones simultaneously, being relevant in multiple ways to the palpation and symptom presentation of the patient. Here are some suggestions for starting points to release the back.

- Du Zone (Includes Huatuo Jiaji lines)
    - Essential Point: Du 17
        - Support point Du 14
            - Additional support point is SI 3, use ipsilateral SI 3 for any lingering tenderness along Huatuo Jiaji points. Frequently used for scoliosis
                - If someone has shoulder Small Intestine channel problems and had Du channel tenderness, maybe choose SI 3 first
- Bladder (inner and outer lines) Zone
    - Essential Point: BL 9
        - BL 62 is support point
            - The exception to this is if pain shows up primarily at the Kidney Zone BL 51-52
                - Then support point is Kd 6
- Gall Bladder Zone
        - (mostly hip area) – This is often ASIS, piriformis and IT band
        - also Dai Mai and ASIS/ilium/groin
    - Essential Point - Du 17 and/or BL 9
        - If IT band
            - GB 26 as support point
        - If piriformis muscle (GB 30 area)
            - GB 25 as support point
        - If Sacrum area or sciatic pain which runs down the entire leg
            - Use Huatuo Jiaji of L5

If anything still left over, use GB 41 or GB 25. For patients who complain of a lot of physical or mental stress as part of chief complaint, use GB 25.

If a few spots left over or just one individual little spot, then use GB 41.

ACU-ZONE TREATMENT PART 1: ESSENTIAL TREATMENT

No matter what the disease may be, acupuncture treatment begins from here. If you choose the right point, you can reduce pain or tenderness anywhere on the body.

There are two approaches – Yin Essential Points, which broadly influence the anterior aspect of the body, and Yang Essential Points, which broadly influence the posterior aspect of the body. Typically treatment is only given to one side during a session, and I prioritize the side on which a patient's chief complaint and/or tenderness to palpation are dominant.

Yin Essential Points

These are Yin Tang (Hall of Impression), bilateral BL 2 (Gathered Bamboo) and Tai Yang (Great Yang).

Yang Essential Points

These are comprised of three points: Du 17 (Brain's Door), BL 9 (Jade Pillow) and GB 12 (Mastoid Process).

Essential Points are chosen based on zone palpation. Tenderness of the treatment points is not desired. These points are never palpated for the most tender spot in an area, they are found by gently palpating for a small depression.

Yin Tang – Hall of Impression

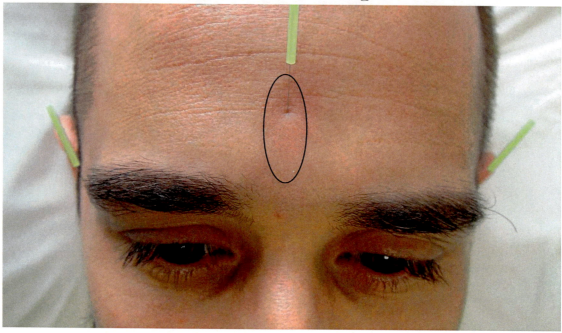

Location: On the ventral midline, best found by palpating gently down the Du Channel from Du 24 towards the space between the eyebrows, where your finger stops in a small depression.

Note: This point is considered to be in this area, there is no precise point location to describe. Each person will be different.

Technique: #03 needle (0.10x15mm). Oblique insertion, .1-.2 *cun* depth, downward with the flow of the Ren Meridian. Synergetic Qi needle technique.

Indication: mainly functions to relieve either the tenderness upon palpation of the Ren Channel, or the patients complaints are along the channel.

A CLINICAL MANUAL OF PRACTICAL ORIENTAL MEDICINE

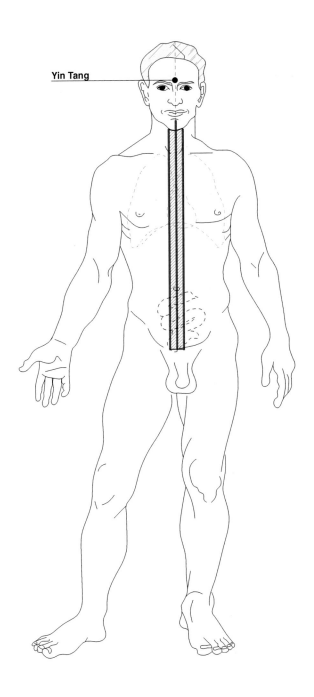

BL 2 – Gathered Bamboo

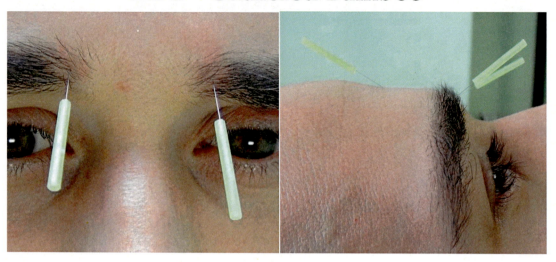

Location: in the depression at the medial end of the eyebrow in the incisura frontalis.

Technique: #03 needle (0.10x15mm). Oblique insertion, .1-.2 *cun* depth, towards BL3, with the flow of the meridian. Synergetic Qi needle technique.

Indications: alleviate pressure pain and symptom in the zone of Kidney Meridian, Spleen Meridian, Liver Meridian, and Stomach Meridian which cover the anterior aspect of the trunk, and between BL10 and BL11.

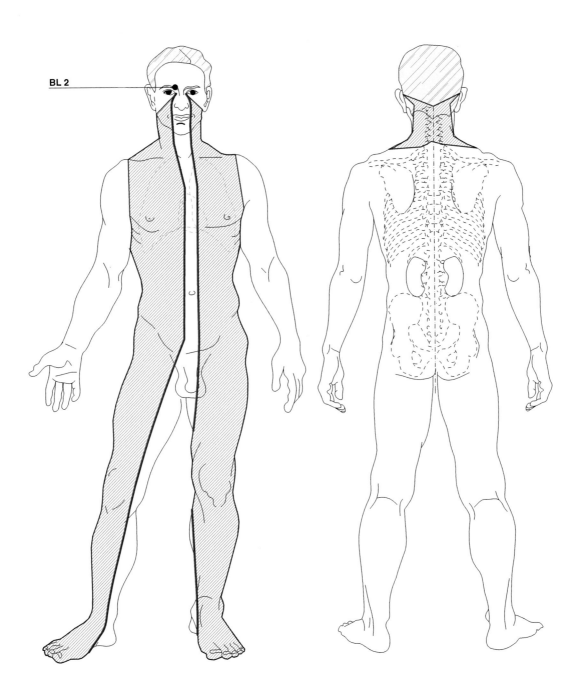

Tai Yang – Great Yang

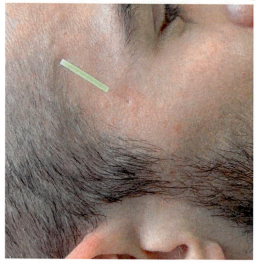

Location: in the depression at the lateral end of the eyebrow, near the bony limit of the orbit.

Technique: #03 needle (0.10x15mm). Oblique insertion, .1-.2 *cun* depth, towards the ipsilateral SCM. Synergetic Qi needle technique.

Indications: Includes lateral aspect of head and neck and anterior aspect of the shoulder, alleviate tenderness and symptoms of Large Intestine, Stomach, and Sanjiao Meridians on the neck and anterior shoulder area, including the SCM muscle.

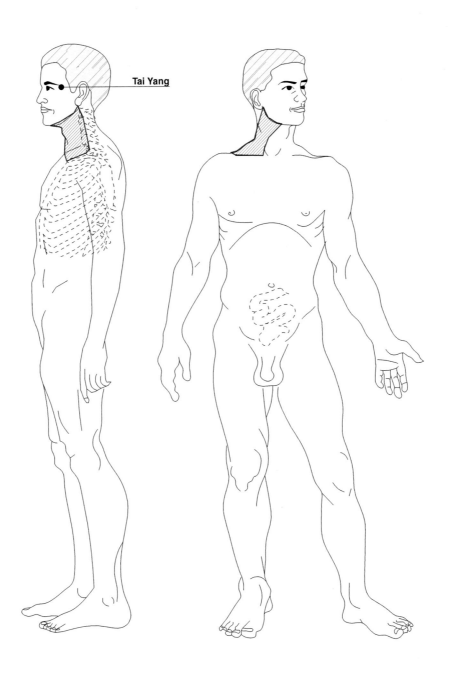

Du 17 – Brain's Door

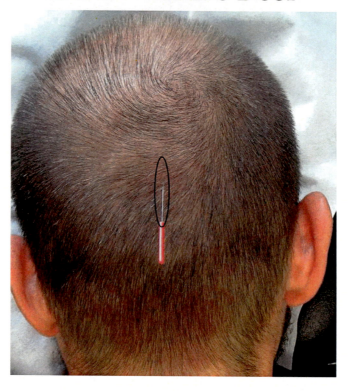

Location: On the dorsal midline, between 1 and 2 *cun* superior to Du 16, at a small depression at the superior border of the external occipital protuberance.

Technique: #1 needle (0.16x30mm), between .1-.3 *cun* depth, oblique insertion, towards Du 20 with the flow of the channel. Synergetic Qi needle technique.

Indication: eases pain along the Du Channel along the spinal column, as well as pain of Huatuo Jiaji points and paraspinal muscles.

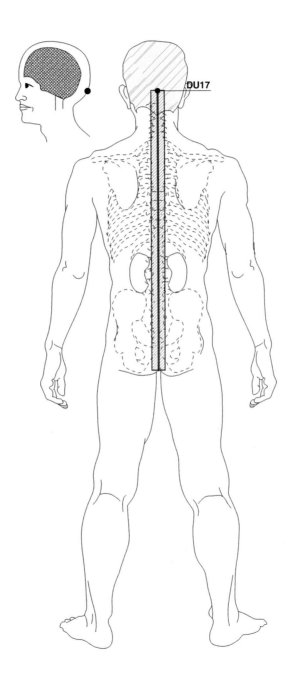

BL 9 – Jade Pillow

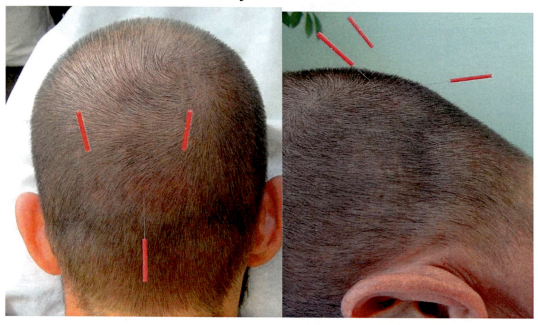

Location: In the area at the level of Du 17, about .5 *cun* lateral to the midline. Palpate for a depression. *Point is selected ipsilaterally to the side of the body that presents with pain upon palpation.*

Technique: #1 needle (0.16x30mm), between .1-.3 *cun* depth, oblique insertion, angled down towards BL 10 with the flow of the Bladder channel. Synergetic Qi needle technique between 10 and 20 seconds, returning to palpate to search for changes, no more than 30 seconds.

Indications: reduces pressure pain along the inner and outer lines of the Bladder Meridian and bottom of feet.

A CLINICAL MANUAL OF PRACTICAL ORIENTAL MEDICINE

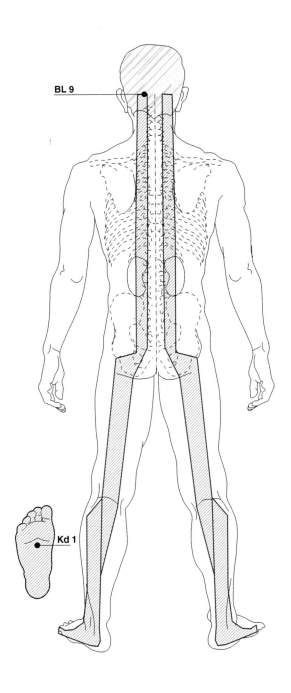

GB 12 – Mastoid Process

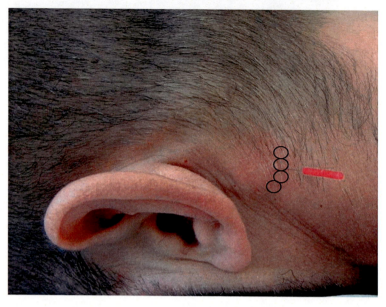

Location: Inferior to the mastoid process. The process is palpated in a "U" shape from all angles towards the process, looking for the most tender location. *Point is selected ipsilaterally to the side of the body that presents with pain upon palpation.*

Technique: #1 needle (0.16x30mm), between .2-.5 *cun* depth, needled very close to the bone, perpendicularly at the location which was most tender on palpation. Synergetic Qi needle technique.

Indication: reduces the tenderness along and diseases of Sanjiao, Small Intestine, Large Intestine, Pericardium, Heart, and Lung Meridians (all meridians of the arm), including shoulder, arm and hand. Also includes pain along Gallbladder Meridian and includes the buttocks and legs.

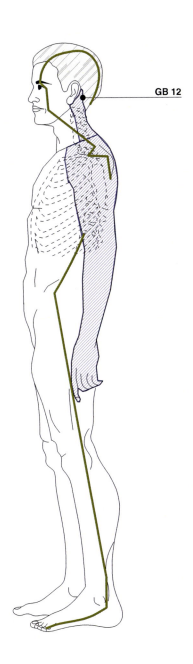

ACU-ZONE TREATMENT PART 2: SUPPORT TREATMENT

These points are utilized with great frequency in combination with the Essential points. They are the second phase of treatment if the patient is lying prone or on their side, or, in the case of the final "touch-up" phase of the treatment, when they are sitting or standing. This phase happens once you have clarified the treatment by using the appropriate Essential Points.

After needling and stimulating the Essential point(s) a good deal of the patient's pain and tenderness in the evaluation zones of the back, neck and adjacent areas should clear up. If the patient presented with pain or tenderness along multiple zones, theoretically the correct selection and location of the Essential point should leave us with a much simpler presentation of pain – usually along just one or two channels or in just a few single spots. In this way it will be easier for us to continue to select just a few points that serve to cover multiple areas, internally as well as externally, simultaneously.

If multiple points in a certain zone show up, or a large zone, we will select the Support points. If there is only one tender spot left or pain along just one channel, we will select the Synthesis point, discussed in the next chapter. Think about the treatment like peeling an onion – removing layers at a time.

Huatuo Jiaji at the level of L5 (HJL5)

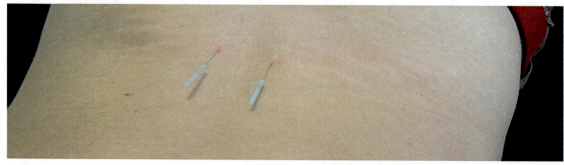

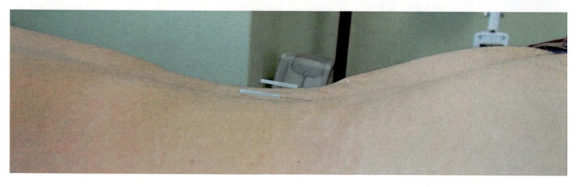

Location: The depression below the spinous process of L5, 0.5-1 *cun* lateral to the dorsal midline.

Technique: any #3 needle (0.20x40mm) or in the case of an obese patient, (0.25x50mm) 1.5~2 *cun* oblique (30~45 degrees) in a downward direction. Synergetic Qi needle technique for about 10 - 20 seconds. If cold lower extremities, apply foot sauna.

Indications: Any disease of the lower limbs, especially the knee and the sole of the foot disorders and sciatica. Also for pain, stiffness, or disorders affecting the area along the cervical vertebrae to the occipital region at the BL 10.

The points have been selected by looking at the primary meridians as well as the Sinew channels of the Bladder, Gall Bladder , and Stomach, Spleen, Kidney, Liver for lower limb meridians – i.e. everything under L5 vertebrae. We can use these Jiaji points for any symptoms that show up in those zones.

A CLINICAL MANUAL OF PRACTICAL ORIENTAL MEDICINE

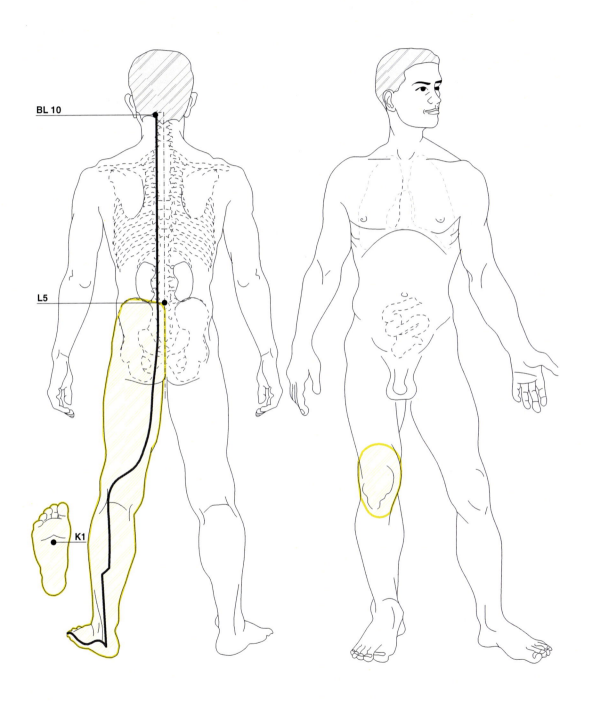

Kd 1 – Bubbling Spring

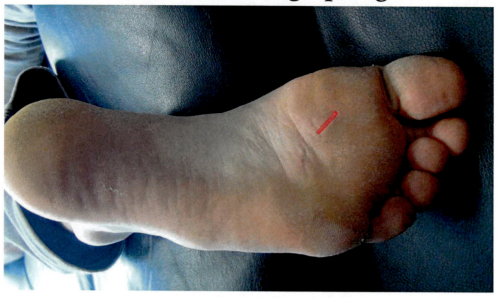

Location: With the foot plantar flexed, in the depression formed in the sole. Same as the TCM location.

Technique: Japanese #03 needle (0.10x15mm).
0.5~1 *cun* oblique (15~45 degrees) with the flow of the meridian, unless symptoms are at toes, in which case the needle should be angled toward the affected toes. For heel pain, the needle can also be directed towards the area of pain. If cold feet, apply the foot sauna. Synergetic Qi needle technique.

Indications: heel pain, plantar fasciitis, pain at the dorsum of the foot, neuropathy, calf cramps, as well as disorders of the head such as headache (especially heat in the head) and menopause symptoms such as hot flashes.

A CLINICAL MANUAL OF PRACTICAL ORIENTAL MEDICINE

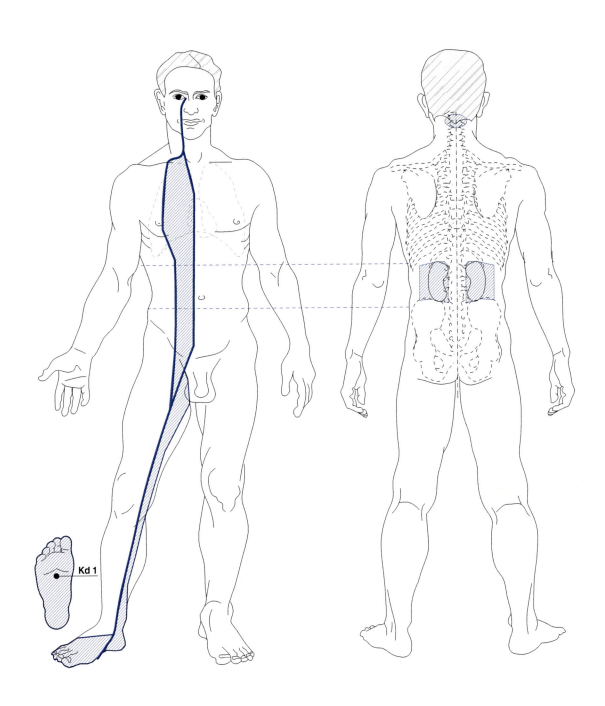

GB 26 – Belt Channel

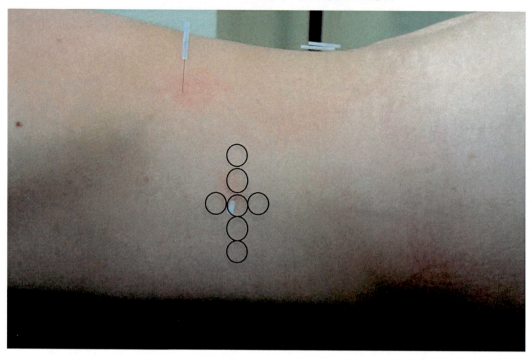

Location: at the intersection of a vertical line through the free end of the 11th rib, and a horizontal line through the umbilicus. This could be found at the halfway point between the highest point of the ilium and the tip of the 11th rib.

This point is found in this area, which can vary greatly depending on the body shape of the individual patient. Palpation at this point may even be quite deep if the patient is obese. The center is at the location described above, and this is where you will begin palpation, searching for a tender or tight spot in the muscle or fascia and below the subcutaneous tissue.

Technique: #3 needle (36 gauge .20x40mm), or in the case of obese patients, perhaps a #5 needle (32 gauge .25x50mm). Depth of 1.5-2 *cun*, perpendicular insertion. Synergetic Qi needle technique for 10-20 seconds.

Indications: Gall Bladder Meridian or Sinew Channel pain. Any pain on the lateral aspect of the body. Can be effective in cases of shoulder pain where it is difficult to raise the arm and tenderness is present along the lateral ribcage. Sciatic pain is also a very common indication. Migraine headache, especially behind the eye. Note: this point can be used in any position that the patient is comfortable – prone, supine, side-lying, sitting, or standing.

A CLINICAL MANUAL OF PRACTICAL ORIENTAL MEDICINE

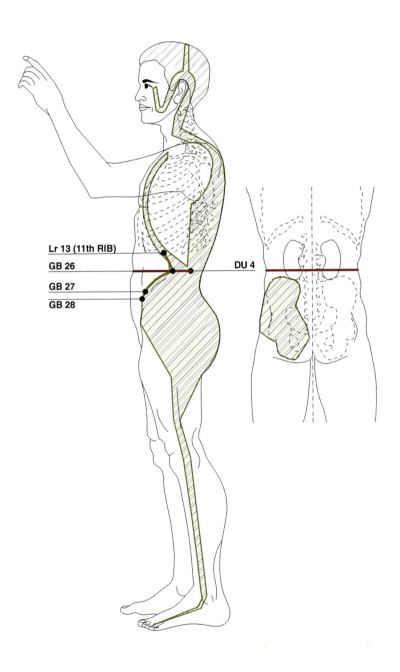

GB 25 – Essence Gate

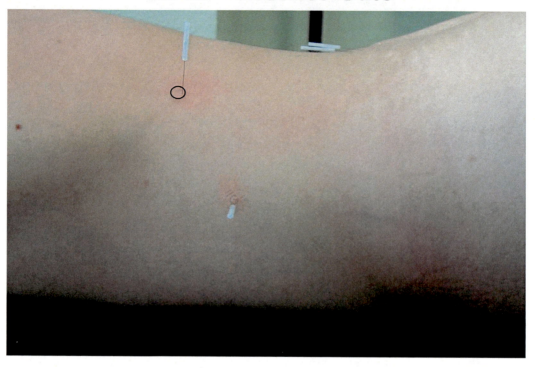

Location: On the inferior border of the free end of the 12th rib.

Technique: #3 needle (36 gauge .20x40mm), or in the case of obese patients, perhaps a #5 needle (32 gauge .25x50mm). Depth of 1.5-2 *cun*, perpendicular insertion. Synergetic Qi needle technique.

Indications: Any Kidney deficiency signs (Yin, Yang, or *qi*), i.e. chronic fatigue, overwork, prolonged mental or physical stress, etc. Any chronic pain or disease case may benefit from the addition of this point at the end of the treatment. This is the only point in the system that is not necessarily chosen by palpation. From clinical experience, the addition of this point seems to help the effects of acupuncture treatments to last longer, especially in chronic cases.

This point may also help release Bladder meridian and sinew zones.

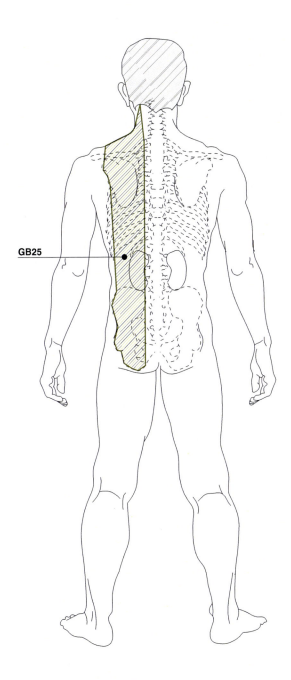

Du 14 – Great Vertebra

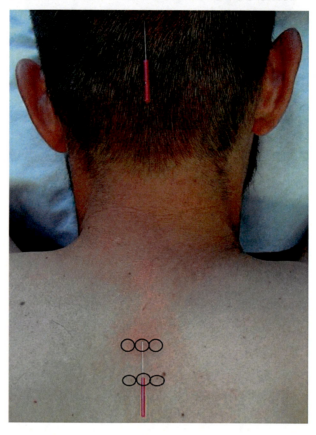

Location: On the dorsal midline in the depression below the spinous process of C7. (*Note*: Du 13, which is located below the spinous process of T1, is also commonly palpated. The more tender of the two points is the one selected for treatment) It can be located on either side of central location, look for it based on pain location.

Technique: Japanese #1 needle (0.16x30mm). Oblique upwards with the flow of the Du channel, depth of .5-1 *cun*, very superficial. Synergetic Qi needle technique.

Indications: Mainly used as a support point for Du 17 when it doesn't completely release the Du channel and there are only one or two spots left. In the post-treatment part of the session, if there is lingering pain at the spine anywhere, Du 14 is needled, briefly stimulated, then removed.

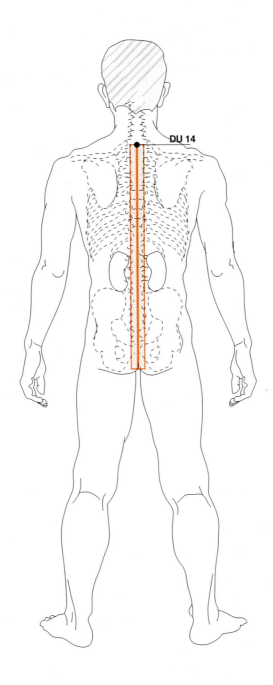

SI 13 – Crooked Wall

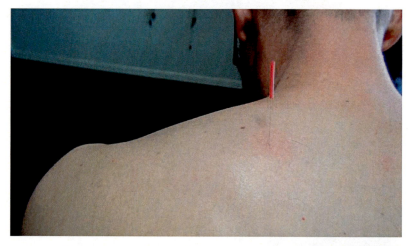

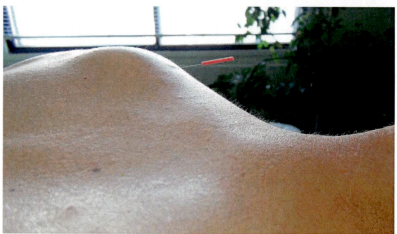

Location: At the medial end of the fossa supraspinata, at the midpoint between SI 10 and the spinous process of T2.

Technique: Japanese #1 needle (0.16x30mm). Oblique insertion down, angled toward the sacro-iliac joint. Synergetic Qi needle technique.

Indications: Symptoms of pain along SI channel, especially along elbow, forearm or hand. Often used as part of the post-treatment final touches, to release any remaining soreness, stiffness, tightness or pain in at the sacro-iliac joint area. Point is needled when standing up, with hands resting on the table.

A CLINICAL MANUAL OF PRACTICAL ORIENTAL MEDICINE

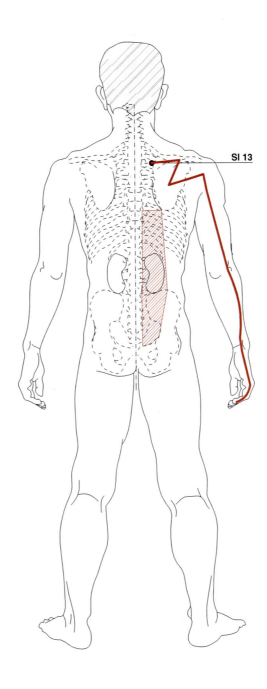

ACU-ZONE TREATMENT PART 3: SYNTHESIS TREATMENT

This is a key part of the concept of looking at the body in terms of zones.

These points come mostly from the opening points of the Eight Extraordinary Meridians, but I added four more points. By weaving the maps of the Extraordinary, Primary, Divergent, and Sinew Meridians together, I have come up with an integrated system which is comprised of just 12 points used to address the entire body.

After palpation of the abdomen, neck, back or painful/tender areas, we carefully mark all tender spots. This guides us to the broad zones. Essential Points are used first in order to clear the majority of tenderness in the zones, and any remaining zones are treated with the Synthesis Points.

Lu 7 – Broken Sequence

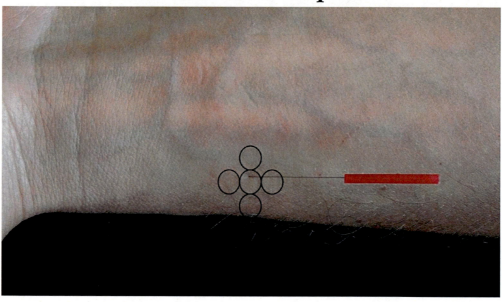

Location: The point is found by starting with the finger at Lu 9 and sliding it towards Lu 5, along the Lung Channel. The point is found in a depression, at a tender area, usually about 1-2 *cun* proximal to Lu 9.

Technique: #03 needle (0.10x15mm), 0.3~0.5 *cun* transverse with the flow of the meridian. Synergetic Qi needle technique for about 10~20 seconds until reduction of the symptom or tenderness.

Indications: Lung diseases such as coughing, shortness of breath, cold/flu symptoms (External Pathogenic Factor), sore throat, and Lung zone (Lu 1 or Lu 2 tenderness), support point for Yin Tang point to release Ren Channel tenderness. Can be used to reduce tenderness at the ipsilateral SCM and Jian Qian area. Also, tenderness or pain at the BL 13-42 area.

A CLINICAL MANUAL OF PRACTICAL ORIENTAL MEDICINE

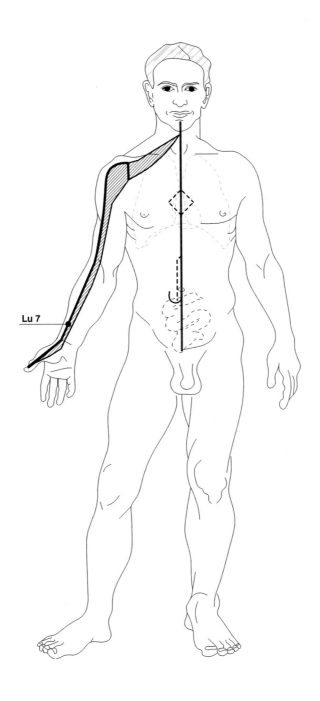

LI 4 – Joining Valley

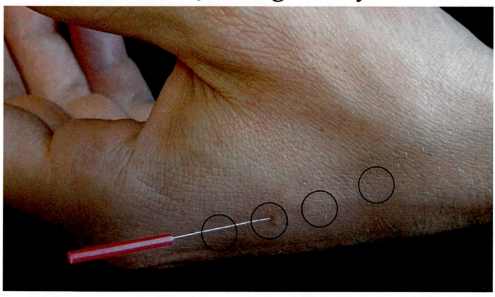

Location: on the dorsum of the hand, in an area beginning at LI 3 and extending proximally along the side of the second metacarpal bone. The area is divided into four divisions, and palpated along the bone for a tender spot.

Technique: #03 needle (0.10x15mm), 0.3~0.5 *cun* transverse with the flow of the meridian. Synergetic Qi needle technique for about 10~20 second until reduction of the symptom or tenderness.

Indication: Large Intestine meridian symptoms (elbow, shoulder, neck, face), especially brachial plexus reflex point. Occasionally used as a support point for LI Zone tenderness. Also, tenderness or pain at the ST 25 area.

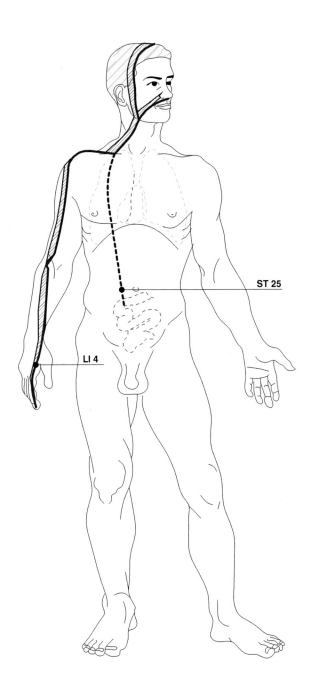

ST 43 – Sunken Valley/Outer ST 43

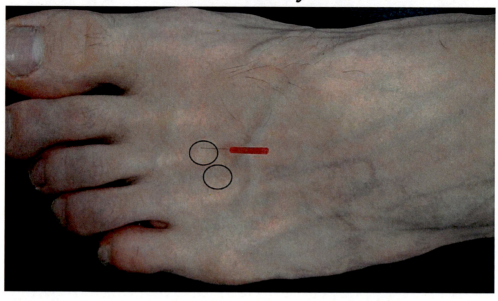

Location: in the depression in the proximal corner of the second metatarso-phalangeal joint, between the second and third toes. Palpate for tenderness. A second area is palpated just laterally to this point, betweem the third and fourth toes. The more tender of the two points is selected for treatment.

Technique: #03 needle (0.10x15mm), 0.3~0.5 *cun* transverse with the flow of the meridian. Synergetic Qi needle technique for about 10~20 seconds until reduction of the symptom or tenderness.

Indications: TMJ, Brachial plexus, sinus pressure, Stomach Meridian issues (knee pain along channel, pain or tenderness along meridian on abdomen). Also, tenderness or pain at the BL 21-50 area.

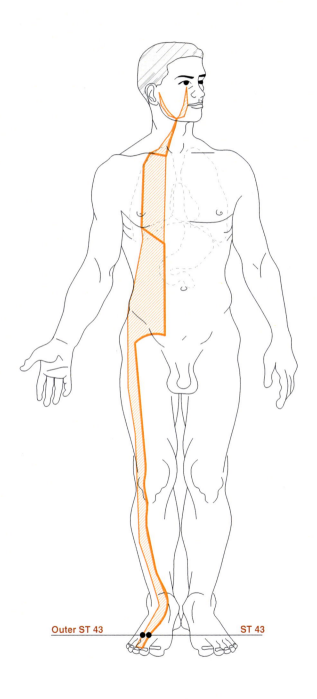

Sp 4 – Grandfather Grandson

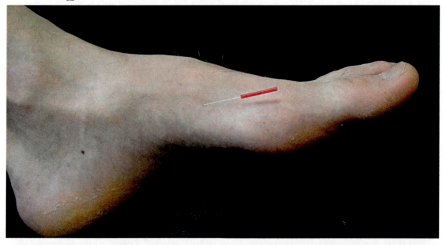

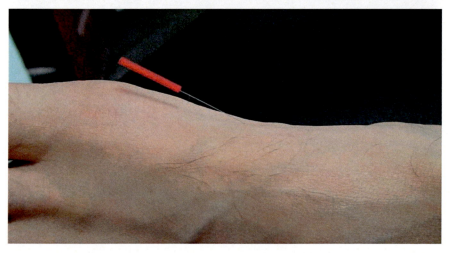

Location: in the depression, distal and inferior to the base of the first metatarsal bone, at the dividing line between red and white flesh

Technique: #03 needle (0.10x15mm), 0.3~0.5 *cun* transverse with the flow of the meridian. Synergetic Qi needle technique for about 10~20 second until reduction of the symptom or tenderness.

Indications: Spleen Zone and also left side of C3 vertebra tenderness. If Ren 15-10 tenderness is not first resolved with Yin Tang, Sp 4 is the support point. If still left over, Pc 6 is used as a secondary support point. Digestive issues, blood sugar imbalances, TCM Spleen organ patterns including gas, bloating, etc., inner knee pain (ipsilateral). Also used for pain or tenderness along Chong Meridian (Sp 4, Sp 6, Kd 10, ST 30, Kd 11, Kd 21, ST 11). Also, tenderness or pain at the BL 20 and 49 area.

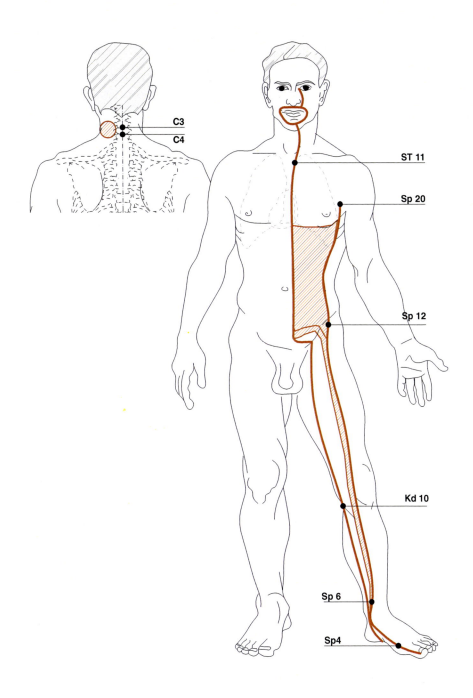

Ht 5 – Penetrating the Interior

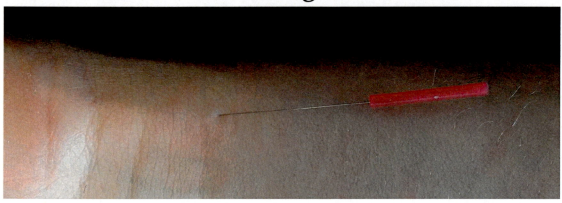

Location: 1 *cun* proximal to the distal wrist crease, on the radial side of the tendon of flexor carpi ulnaris

Technique: #03 needle (0.10x15mm), 0.3~0.5 *cun* transverse with the flow of the meridian. Synergetic Qi needle technique for about 10~20 second until reduction of the symptom or tenderness.

Indications: Heart zone tenderness, physical heart issues such as palpitations, irregular heart beat, left-sided chest pain. Also, tenderness or pain at the BL 15-44 area.

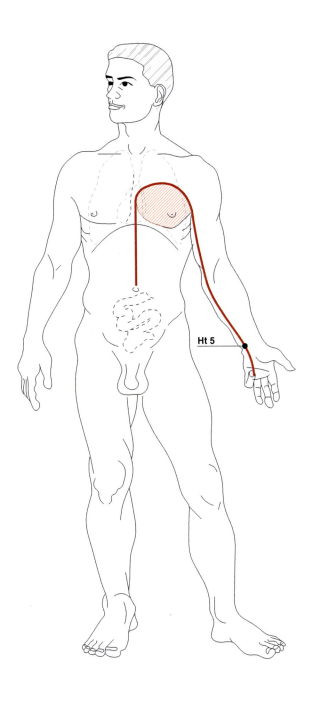

SI 3 – Back Stream

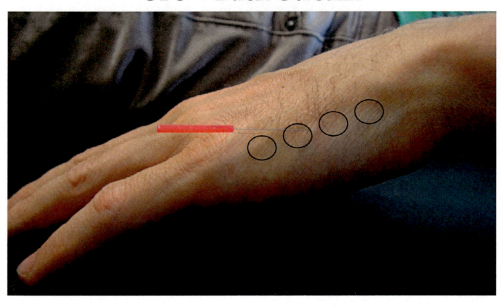

Location: The area on the ulnar side of the palm, beginning from the proximal crease of the fifth metacarpophalangeal joint and going to SI 4 which is the base of the fifth metacarpal bone and triquetral bone. Palpate along the 5th metacarpal bone for the most tender points.

Technique: #03 needle (0.10x15mm), 0.3~0.5 *cun* transverse with the flow of the meridian. Synergetic Qi needle technique for about 10~20 second until relieving the symptom or tenderness.

Indication: Tenderness of the posterior midline from the cervical to lumbar region, along the Du meridian. Any symptom on the small intestine meridian. Also, tenderness or pain at the BL 27 area and Ren 4.

A CLINICAL MANUAL OF PRACTICAL ORIENTAL MEDICINE

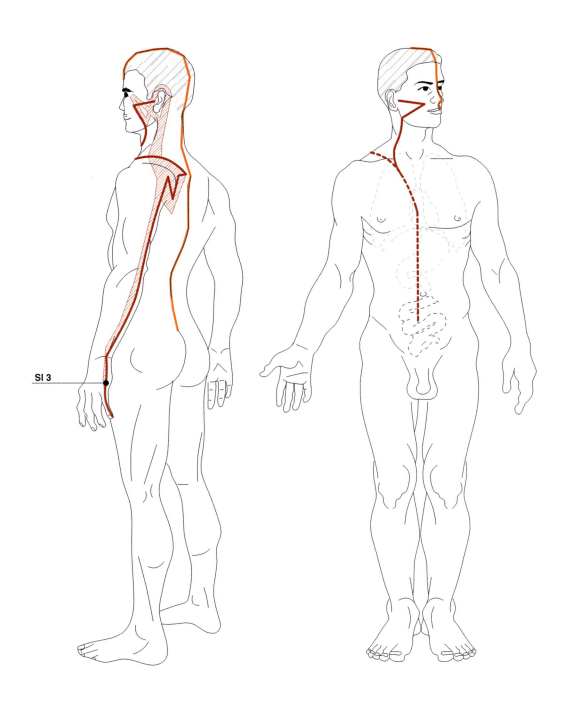

BL 62 – Extending Vessel

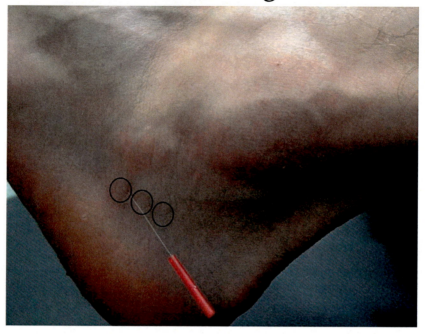

Location: in the depression distal to the lateral malleolus. This area should be carefully palpated, and the most tender spot is needled.

Technique: #03 needle (0.10x15mm), 0.3~0.5 *cun* transverse with the flow of the meridian. Synergetic Qi needle technique for about 10~20 second until reduction of the symptom or tenderness.

Indications: Bladder Meridian and zones, mostly for low back pain and SI joint, pain behind knee, sciatica. Also for pain or tenderness along the Yang Qiao Meridian. Can be used to help with pain at Kidney shu points, between BL 23 and 52. Typically used as a support point. Also, tenderness or pain at the BL 28-53 area.

A CLINICAL MANUAL OF PRACTICAL ORIENTAL MEDICINE

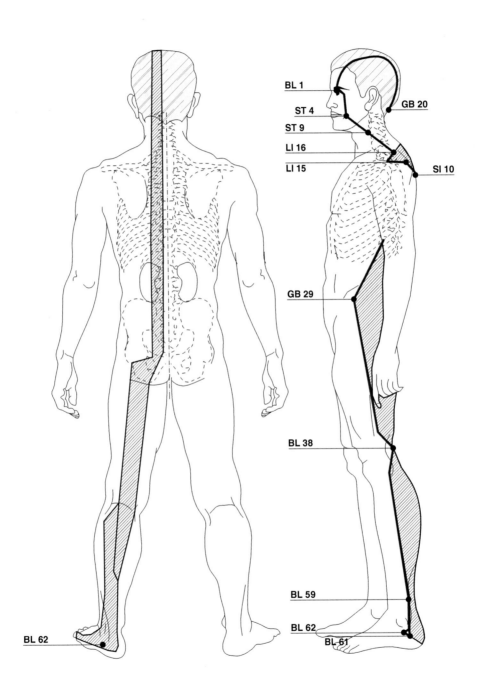

Kd 6 – Shining Sea

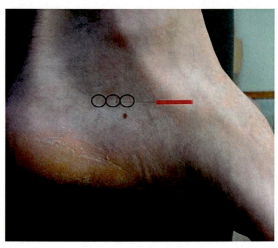
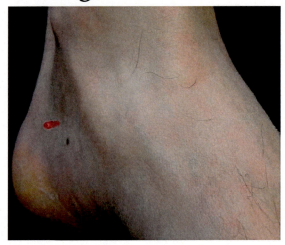

Location: in the depression inferior to the inferior border of the medial malleolus. This area should be carefully palpated, and the most tender spot is needled.

Technique: #03 needle (0.10x15mm), 0.3~0.5 *cun* transverse with the flow of the meridian. Synergetic Qi needle technique for about 10~20 second until reduction of the symptom or tenderness.

Indications: In comparison with BL 62, Kd 6 is used for more internal disorders of Bladder and Kidney, whereas BL 62 is more for "external" issues, such as musculoskeletal issues, etc. Releasing of Kidney/Bladder zones is the most important indicatations for these points. Also used for pain or tenderness along Yin Qiao Meridian(Kd11~27 and ST12~30) and tenderness or pain at the BL 22, 23-51, 52 area.

A CLINICAL MANUAL OF PRACTICAL ORIENTAL MEDICINE

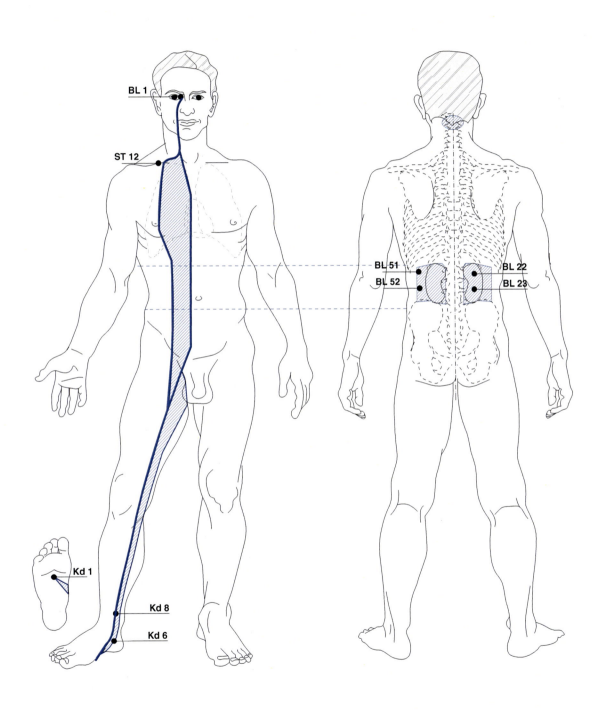

Pc 6 – Inner Gate

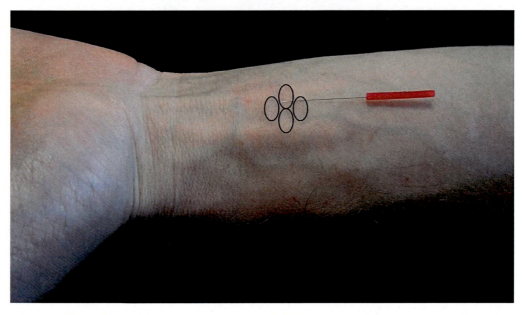

Location: 2 *cun* proximal to the distal wrist crease, on the connecting line between Pc 3 and Pc 7, between the palmaris longus and flexor carpi radialis tendons. *For internal conditions, palpation of a tender spot is not necessary.* In conditions of pain in the hand or fingers, palpate for the most tender spot.

Technique: #03 needle (0.10x15mm), 0.3~0.5 *cun* transverse with the flow of the meridian. Synergetic Qi needle technique for about 10~20 second until reduction of the symptom or tenderness.

Indications: Pericardium zone on the abdomen, emotional issues, such as anxiety, nervousness, insomnia, emotionally-related digestion issues. Used as a secondary point for alleviating the tendernss on SCM #3 with heart symtoms. For pain or tenderness along Yin Wei Meridian(Kd 9, Kd 10, Sp 10, Sp 13, Lr 14, Ren 17, Ren 23). Also, tenderness or pain at the BL 14-43 area and Kd 10 area knee pain.

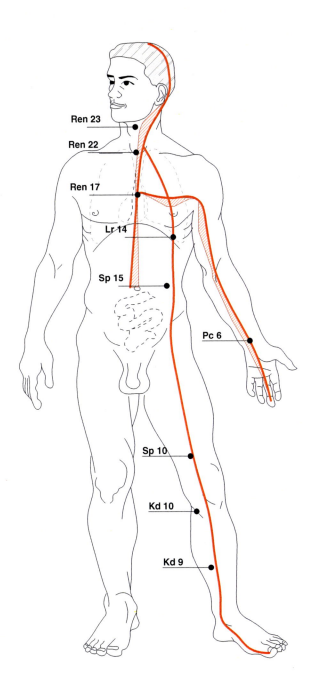

SJ 5 – Outer Gate

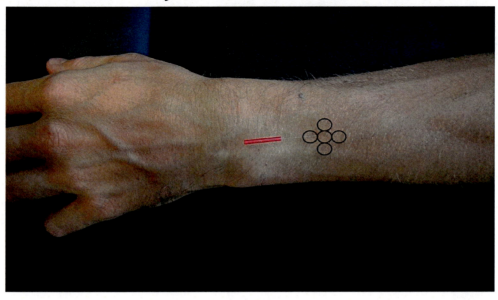

Location: 2 *cun* distal to the dorsal wrist crease between the ulna and radius

Technique: #03 needle (0.10x15mm), 0.3~0.5 *cun* transverse with the flow of the meridian. Synergetic Qi needle technique for about 10~20 second until reduction of the symptom or tenderness.

Indications: SCM muscle tenderness or lymphatic issues, neck/shoulder/ear pain along San Jiao channel. Pain or tenderness along Yang Wei Meridian.

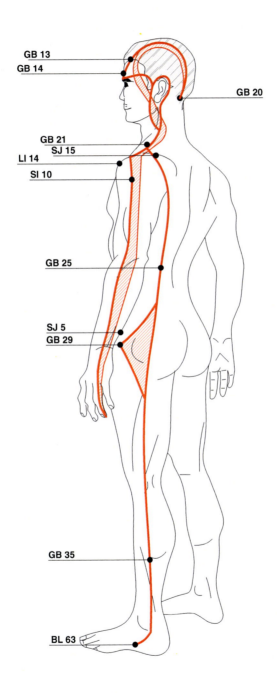

GB 41 – Foot Governor of Tears / GB 42 – Earth Five Meetings

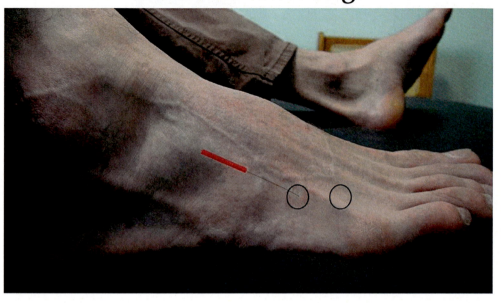

Location: on the dorsum of the foot, between the fourth and fifth metatarsal bones, proximal to the fourth metatarso-phalangeal joint, in the depression medial to the tendon of the extensor digiti minimi longus. These two points, GB 41 and GB 42, are palpated for tenderness. Typically it is GB 42 that is more tender, and often the first choice for palpation, but both should be carefully checked and the most tender is the appropriate treatment point.

Technique: #03 needle (0.10x15mm), 0.3~0.5 *cun* transverse with the flow of the meridian. Synergetic Qi needle technique for about 10~20 second until reduction of the symptom or tenderness.

Indications: Commonly used for Gall Bladder meridian pain such as headache, hip, sciatic nerve pain, outer knee, GB 21 tension, tenderness along Dai Meridian including GB 26 and the line around waist at level of Du 4, as well as along the ASIS at GB 27 and 28. Also, tenderness or pain at the BL 19-48 area.

A CLINICAL MANUAL OF PRACTICAL ORIENTAL MEDICINE

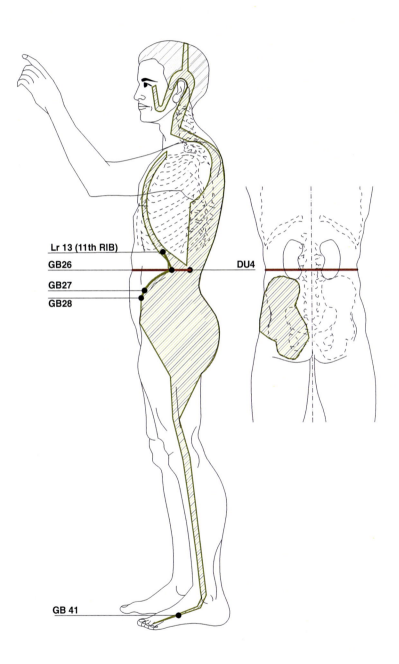

Lr 3 – Great Rushing

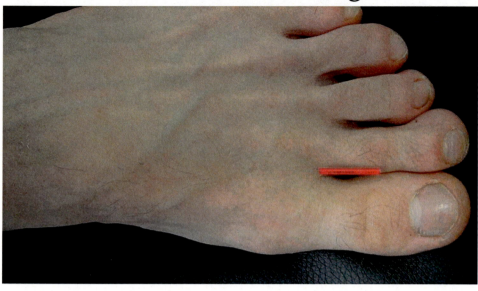

Location: on the dorsum of the foot, in the depression distal to the proximal corner between the first and second metatarsal bones

Technique: #03 needle (0.10x15mm), 0.3~0.5 *cun* transverse with the flow of the meridian. Synergetic Qi needle technique for about 10~20 second until reduction of the symptom or tenderness.

Indications: Liver zone and right-sided abdominal complaints, as well as right side of C3 vertebra pain. Pain along Liver Meridian, including knee, groin, and eyes. Also, tenderness or pain at the BL 18-47 area.

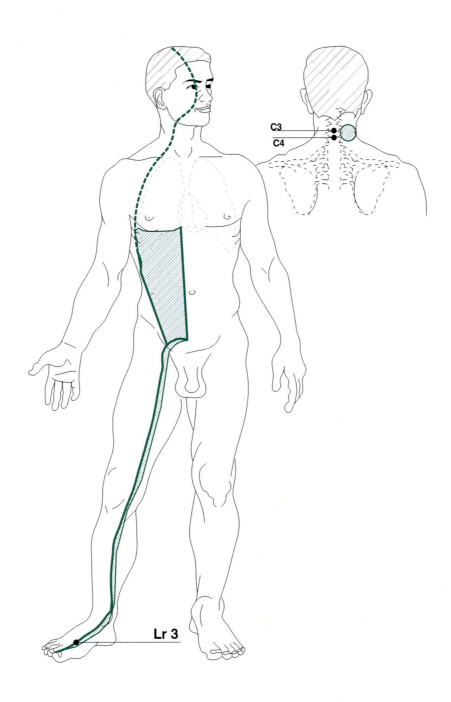

IMPORTANCE OF THE BRAIN STEM: A WESTERN MEDICAL PERSPECTIVE

Why Begin with Essential Points?

Here, I intend to explain the process of internal brain function when acupuncture needles are inserted at Essential Points. With it, you will better understand how my treatment style works, and also why I focus on the use of these points. In short, the Essential Points activate the brainstem's neural network and restores homeostasis. The return to homeostasis results in self-healing. With this core belief in the self-healing mechanism, I propose a practical working theory of how Integrated Synergy Therapeutics works.

Basic Concept: Brainstem

Here is a list of the brainstem's physiological responsibilities:

- Autonomic Nervous system regulation: Rest/Digest, fight/flight
- Circulatory regulation: Blood pressure, volume
- Eliminatory regulation: Urination, defecation, perspiration
- Primordial desire regulation: Appetite, reproduction and libido, sleep
- Thermoregulation : Sweating, temperature control
- Immuno-modulation: Fighting and preventing infections and invasions
- Emotional Regulation: Stress, perception, psychological stability
- Motor and Sensory Communication
- Postural Reflex: Postural and balance control

Although the brain stem comprises only 5% of our brain, it is what allows us to heal ourselves and coordinate non-stop function and regulation of our vital organs. The twelve cranial nerves serve as a communication bridge between sensory and motor organs and the interpretive center of the brain. I propose that effective acupuncture treatment influences this communication bridge. Then with proper stimulation and guidance, the body heals better through visceral-somatic, somato-viceral, and somato-somatic connections.

Acupuncture Theory with Brainstem and Cranial Nerves

1: Vagus Nerve and Spinal Accessory Nerve: Acupuncture utilizes visceral and somatic connections.

The 10th cranial nerve, i.e the vagus nerve, innervates the abdomen and the organs through to the transverse colon via sensory and motor nerves within the parasympathetic nervous system.

Ren 15 is where the major plexus is located and has 10 branches from that point:

1. Hepatic Plexus 2. Splenic Plexus 3. Gastric Plexus 4. Pancreatic Plexus 5. Suprarenal Plexus 6. Renal Plexus 7. Testicular/Ovarian Plexus 8. Superior Mesenteric Plexus 9. Inferior Mesenteric Plexus 10. Celiac Plexus

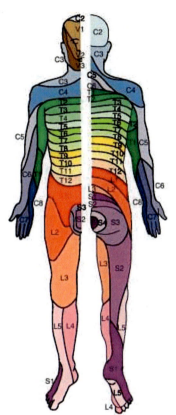

Each organ exhibits a referral zone at a certain surface location. These are called visceral-somatic reflexes. It is a phenomenon of the body communicating the information of organs to the brain and at the same time relaying the information in pain form to the skin surface/muscle fibers via the shared spinal cord location between sensory nerves and motor nerves. Conversely, the phenomenon that skin surface stimulation influences the internal organs is called somato-visceral reflexes. This is a main avenue where acupuncture is accessing and influencing the tension and pain of internal organs and muscles via needles and moxibustion. In the same manner, the stimulation of the skin goes to the shared spinal nerves and plexus of certain organs, therefore affecting more than just skin, but the organs that share the same nerve. This would result in more blood flow and homeostasis of organ system functions. Osteopathy had developed this idea and utilizes the same mechanisms for explaining how some Osteopathic Manipulative Treatments work. In addition, the spread of each spinal nerve's connection to skin is shown in the dermatome diagram to the left.

By applying this knowledge, one could search for an associated organ and/or system problem with any muscular pain. Since the brain stem controls the postural reflex system (which controls the tension and relaxation of the spine and limbs), the use of Essential Points automatically releases constriction of muscles via the nerves.

The eleventh cranial nerve, the spinal accessory nerve, runs via the medulla oblongata into the spinal cord. Once coming out of the spinal cord, it joins with the 3rd and 4th cervical nerves, innervating the sternocleidomastoid muscle and trapezius muscle. One coming out of medulla oblongata joins with the vagus nerve then innervates the same muscle group. By relaxing this muscle group, an acupuncturist can easily guide the body from sympathetic nervous mode to the parasympathetic nervous mode. Achieving good balance of the autonomic nervous system, brain and body so that it can communicate smoothly.

This is the very reason why I strongly emphasize the reduction of tightness and pain at the sternocleidomastoid and trapezius muscle. I hope readers can understand the importance of the abdominal diagnosis and the cervical diagnosis. They serve as a window into the current state of the patient's autonomic nervous system.

2: Sore muscle and cranial nerves

Here, I explain the most intriguing aspect of my treatment style: instant pain relief. You must understand how the pain is communicated to the brain first. Initially, the pain that was perceived at the receptor is converted to the electric pulse/signal. The electric signal reaches the spinal cord via nervous root ganglia through nerves. In the spinal cord, the electric signal becomes a neurotransmitter. The neurotransmitter is sorted and relayed to the brain. In the brain, the signal is sent to the cerebral cortex and limbic system where it is interpreted as pain.

The pain signal excites two types of pain control after the information sent via the spinal cord reaches the brainstem. One is the descending modulation of the pain. It controls the pain by regulating the synaptic transmission between the primary nociceptive neuron of the posterior horn of the spinal cord, and a secondary nociceptive neuron from the brainstem by inhibitory interneurons. Noradrenaline from the brainstem and serotonin from the medulla oblongata act to down-regulate the pain perception. Another type of pain control comes via the endogenic opioid substance from the hypothalamus. When opioid receptors receive a stimulus (ex., β-endorphins, enkephalins, dynorphins, etc.), the pain is alleviated by either preventing neurotransmitter release by lowering calcium ion influx into the presynaptic terminal, or by opening potassium channels to hyperpolarize neurons and down-regulate the spike.

Then, how is it that the mechanical stimulation of acupuncture works for relieving pain? Acupuncture needles stimulate the A-delta fibers and C fibers at the polymodal nociception center on the skin, resulting in descending modulation of pain. The axons of A-delta fibers transmit pain rapidly and the C fibers transmit it slowly. By stimulating the nociceptive mechanisms without causing a lot of pain using sharp and painless needles, patients can feel the pain relief at the various body parts. Pain control via the Diffuse Noxious Inhibitory Control system by stimulating organs, skin, and, muscles may share similar mechanisms to how acupuncture induces inhibitory interneurons. Now, why are there so many chronic pain patients even though we have such strong pain regulating mechanisms in our bodies?

3: Sources of chronic pain - Stress can control pain short-term but can worsen pain long-term.

Acute stress pain relief mechanism.

When the body feels acute stress, it activates the hypothalamus and the sympathetic nervous system becomes predominant, releasing noradrenaline and catecholamine from the medulla of the adrenal glands. These substances can act as pain relievers. Secondly, the hypothalamus can activate the pituitary gland, releasing adrenocorticotropic hormone (ACTH) and beta endorphins. ACTH can stimulate the adrenal cortex, releasing an anti-inflammatory substance: cortisol. Beta endorphin can act like an endogenous pain reliever. These are exemplified by how athletes are capable of continuing playing in the event of injuries. Some would call it "runner's high".

I would like to stress here that the enjoyment of the activity results in release of these substances within the body. Thus, it is ever more important that our patients receive acupuncture treatment in the least painful and most peaceful fashion. I believe that uncomfortable acupuncture sessions can often result in a worse state of pain as opposed to pain relief. Please be mindful of this.

Pain caused by chronic stress.

As pain continues, the sympathetic nervous system goes into overdrive, resulting in poor circulation to muscles and organs, leaving them with less blood and oxygen. In this deprived state muscles contract, resulting in constriction of blood/lymph vessels and nerves. At the same time, the pituitary gland releases vasopressin, resulting in angiotensin being released from the kidneys. This would further constrict blood vessels causing more pain. Sustained sympathetic nervous system drive causes insomnia, increased blood pressure, elevated glucose, fatigue, and frequent virus infection, inducing more stress along the way.

When pain is perceived as stress in the body, the hypothalamus becomes activated increasing sympathetic drive, and releasing more catecholamine. This self-perpetuating cycle with ACTH stimulating the adrenal cortex, results in higher blood pressure and elevated blood glucose.

These reactions are important and essential in "fight or flight" situations, but sustained stress brings on the above described worsened body state. Along with chronic stress, a negative emotional state is far too common. It also contributes to noradrenaline being released and makes the pain receptors more sensitive, creating increased likelihood of chronic pain. Moreover, anxiety, irritation, and insomnia can decrease serotonin levels. Reduction of serotonin would disable the pain control mechanisms in the central nervous system.

Our main job is to liberate patients from the stress of pain via acupuncture as well as to become a good listener in order to find the source of stress and pain for their own recovery.

Above, I endeavored to explain the relationship between pain and Integrated Synergy Therapeutics from a physiological viewpoint including the function of the brainstem. Many experts in the field of neuroscience may disagree with me. However, my focus here is to convey a basic message to the readers: With less than 10 acupuncture points needled with precise location and only gentle vibrations at the needle, you can treat any patient effectively.

WALK-THROUGH OF ACUPUNCTURE TREATMENT

Walk-Through of a Typical Treatment:

The treatment begins with gathering relevant health history and information. You can choose which way you want to gather this, with your own health history forms to help you determine which information is typically pertinent in informing your treatments. The health history doesn't need to be unnecessarily exhaustive, it does need to be comprehensive in that it can give you enough clues to get a global understanding of your patient's condition. For this reason, if a person comes in with a complaint of pain, we know that some traditional questioning can be helpful in narrowing our treatment. Asking about diet, digestion, hot/cold, sleep, elimination, emotional state, etc. are all helpful for us down the road when we will be making our point selection. Eventually, point selection is primarily based on palpation and the release of pain at the evaluation areas, but is guided by our knowledge of the channels and pathologies of the organ systems. There is always a blend of intuition and knowledge here, and a healthy balance needs to happen. In many systems, point selection can be too theoretical. This system is geared toward helping you, the practitioner, be grounded in the reality of the patient yet still be gently guided by theory and your knowledge.

If appropriate, we perform the VEM test in order to determine the correct Chinese herbs or supplements.

Once you have gathered the information needed, you can begin with palpation. If there is pain, begin by exploring the painful zones, obviously taking great care to not cause the person more pain but still be thorough enough to be able to determine exactly the areas where there is pain. Many people are unable to express exactly where the pain is until you begin careful palpation of the area. These areas, specifically the most tender spots, are marked with a non-toxic highlighter directly on the body of the patient. Palpation of the painful areas first is critical for many reasons – one is that we want the patient to know that we are focused on their chief complaint. If we just dive into abdominal palpation when a person comes in for plantar fasciitis, they are confused and begin to wonder what we are doing. Another reason is that since the healing interaction begins once you put your hands on the patient, you are giving a clear message to the body and brain that, "this is where we want to focus healing." Healthy neurological circuiting begins with this. Later we give that pain or disease context in a holistic way by palpating the principle evaluation zones, but for now we want to begin the treatment with this message.

Palpate the area of chief complaint: this will guide you to the Essential point. Our palpation is guided in many ways, and allows us to make numerous connections for the patient's mind and body. We palpate according to

- Meridians
- Nervous pathways (dermatomes)
- Structures (Bones, muscles)
- Internal disorder (organ imbalances)

After the area of primary concern to the patient has been palpated, adjacent areas are also palpated. For example, if a person complains of elbow pain, you may first palpate the elbow for tender points, then check carefully up and down the channels towards the wrist and shoulder for other points. Since the arm is connected to the neck, we will also carefully check the neck and shoulder on that same side and mark tender points. This second phase of palpation of the adjacent areas starts integrating their body and the healing messages are beginning to have a clearer pathway. We eventually want to be able to give the body the simplest message possible. Any area where a patient has pain is the first step, followed by palpation of nearby areas that connect to the trunk or head. Remember, we are thinking in the broadest strokes still at this point. Refinement of the treatment will come much later. We want to move from broadest perspective towards minute detail. Instead of thinking in terms of channels, it may be helpful to think about gross anatomy and dermatomes – the ankle has pain, so I will check nearby areas as well as the hip and low back, because that is the closest junction with the nervous system, and then we can check the neck later. This kind of thinking will allow us to get a broad view first while we are trying to determine the treatment route.

The third phase of palpation involves the principle evaluation zones: the neck, abdomen, and spine. Depending on whether the patient is prone or supine or lateral recumbent you will only palpate either the abdomen or the spine, but always the neck.

Once we have recorded where all the painful areas are which are relevant to the treatment, we begin the process of point selection. Essential points are selected first.

The importance of palpation cannot be overstated. If you watch my clinical videos you will see that I consistently use the same points. You may be tempted to skip the palpation part and jump straight to the needling, but this is not recommended.

A CLINICAL MANUAL OF PRACTICAL ORIENTAL MEDICINE

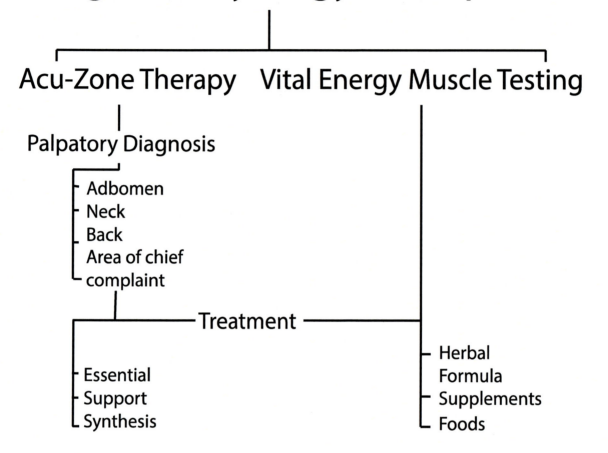

SUPINE:

If most of the tender areas show along the midline, Yin Tang is selected first. If they are more lateral or simply one-sided, either BL 2, Tai Yang, or perhaps even GB 12 is selected. This will depend on your zone analysis.

Once the essential point has been selected, recheck all marked tender spots. If there is any reduction in tenderness at these points or areas, it is likely that you have chosen correctly. If you are palpating and find that there is not a significant reduction in tenderness, either you need to recheck the point location, give a bit more gentle vibrations to the needle, or choose a different Essential point. This is critical for the success of the treatment. Don't be afraid to keep trying. If your point location is correct, you *will* see a marked change in the tender areas.

Once the Essential Point has been needled, the goal is to continue trying to release all remaining painful areas, including that of the chief complaint of the patient as well as the evaluation zones. In the supine position, you will add one or more of the "synthesis points". These points are chosen based on evaluation of the meridian pathways, extraordinary channels, as well as a patient's chief complaint. For example, if a person shows tenderness at the left side of C3 this is typically indicative of a Spleen imbalance. Sp 4 is the point indicated. However, if the patient is also showing tenderness at the left brachial plexus zone, this may be more complicated to diagnose. Many channels pass through this point. How do you decide which is the correct one? Part of that is by palpating surrounding channels, i.e. Large Intestine, Stomach, and Small Intestine. One of these may indicate a tendency towards that channel more than the other. Also, patient's complaints will guide you. How are their bowels? Do they have a low immune system? Is their digestion healthy? These will clue you in to which channel is involved. By palpating the synthesis point of that channel, you should find tenderness. If needled correctly, this should release the remaining tenderness at the point.

The key to point selection is always synthesis. Bringing together the patient's chief complaint, internal condition, knowledge of meridian pathways and nervous system is where the elegant results are found. With enough consideration, only a few needles are selected – I usually use between 2-7 and always fewer than 10.

PRONE and LATERAL RECUMBENT:

Treatment begins with the Essential Point or points. If there is tenderness along the spine or Huatuo Jiajis, then Du 17 is selected and gently stimulated, and then the tender spots rechecked. If the appropriate release of pain was found, treatment can continue. Otherwise, point location should be checked and/or further stimulation is required.

If pain or tenderness is mostly along the Bladder channels or the lower limbs, perhaps BL 9 is a better choice than Du 17. If the issue is on the sides of the body or on the upper limb, GB 12 is the best essential point.

After the selection of the Essential point, the Support Points are the next choice. This is only necessary if there is any tenderness remaining in the zones that you initially palpated. Support points are chosen if larger areas covering multiple channels still remain tender after the Essential Points have been treated.

Lastly we select a Synthesis Point in order to reduce tenderness at any lingering single spots or along one single channel.

A CLINICAL MANUAL OF PRACTICAL ORIENTAL MEDICINE

Select treatment position based on the main complaint or symptoms

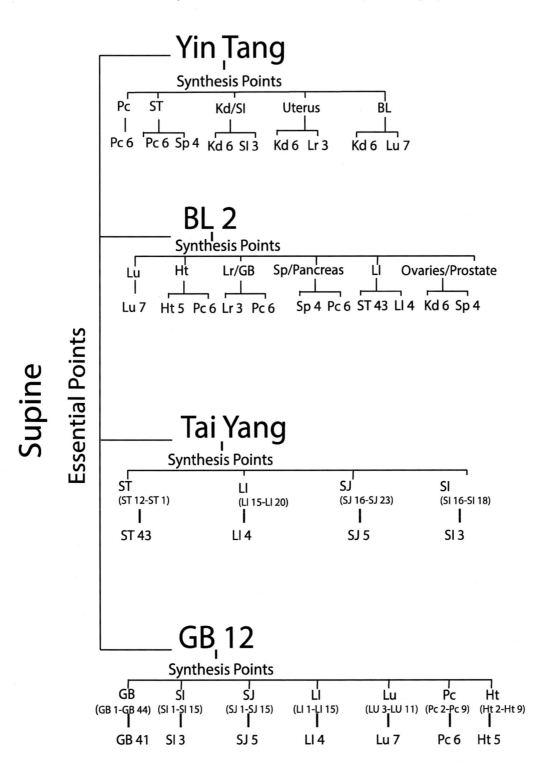

A CLINICAL MANUAL OF PRACTICAL ORIENTAL MEDICINE

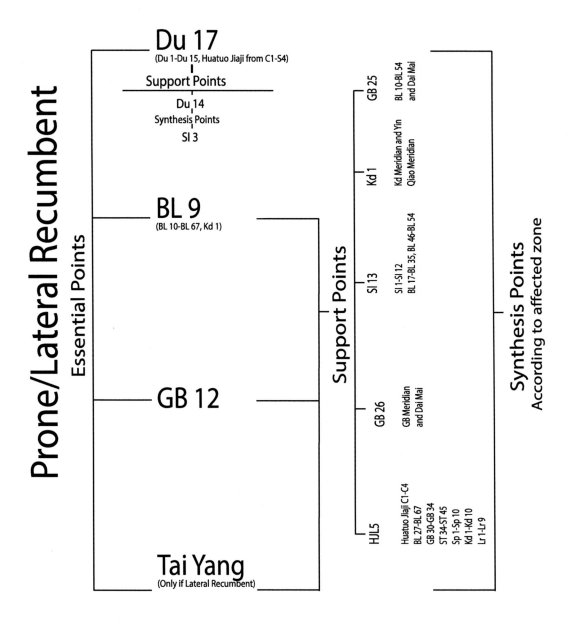

97

VITAL ENERGY MUSCLE (VEM) TESTING

A constant question for us in the clinic is when to make adjustments and when to stay the course. A patient comes in and says, "Things are the same as last week." How do you determine if you need to change your treatment or continue with what you started the previous week?

In general, I believe that acupuncture helps with spontaneous healing and can provide quick relief. I use Chinese herbs as well as supplements to support the treatment and sustain the effects of the acupuncture in order to promote a speedy and full recovery.

In the United States we have an advantage in that we can prescribe herbs and do acupuncture at the same time, not like in Japan. In my practice I try to keep a global perspective when looking at both acupuncture and herbs. The Vital Energy Muscle (VEM) test can really help us hone in on the right formula that will help push the acupuncture treatment to the next level.

VEM testing is beneficial in that it is a way to evaluate which herbs are working, and how effectively. If there are stalls or slow results, the VEM test can determine with more confidence if the person should continue with the formula or if we need to adjust. Also, the VEM test can help us determine which formula and from which company. In my experience, some patents work for some people, while for other people the same formula but just a different company is needed. Even minute adjustments can make all the difference in the world when it comes to progress for a patient.

When starting out prescribing herbs over 20 years ago, I lacked confidence to allow tongue and pulse alone to guide me to the correct formula. Over the years I have developed this system which hopefully will give you another tool in your clinic to be able to arrive at an appropriate herbal formula or supplement for your patients.

VITAL ENERGY MUSCLE TESTING

Vital Energy Muscle Testing is based on the fact that the human body and each substance have their own unique electric and electromagnetic fields. This test detects how a particular substance interacts with the human body and even its individual organs. We can determine if the substance interacts with the body in a positive or negative way.

This method allows us to use the sensitivity of the body, which is capable of detecting even a very faint stimulus. We can check the change in the tonus of a minor muscle to observe how the body reacts to that stimulus. It allows us to work without the use of diagnostic instruments.

CONCEPT OF ENERGY

All substances in reality are composed of vibrating quantum fields. Everything in the cosmos is made of clusters of elementary particles, and life takes distinct shape based on how these clusters interact. Everything is woven together in one inter-linked whole.

The human body is no exception – it is made of the same elementary particles. Clusters of these particles take on different vibrations and create distinct energy fields – such as the hepatic or the nephric energy fields. Looked at as a whole, the human body appears to be one seamless energy field. Viewed more closely it will show the distinct energy fields of each organ.

I believe that life force expresses in ways that are not always visible to the human eye – such as electromagnetic waves, a micro-current, a frequency, a wavelength, a rhythm, a ray of light, and even consciousness. All of these work together to express as life force.

We are alive because the universe gave us resonance power. This is more than a vibration – a vibration implies a solitary wave. Resonance, on the other hand, suggests two or more things communicating.

Stagnation, deficiency, and disharmony of this energy produce the abnormal conditions in the human body – in other words, disease.

SYSTEM OF VITAL ENERGY MUSCLE TESTING

This test can detect any abnormality in the human energy field.

By placing slight pressure on certain areas of the body, we can stimulate a sensory neuron to send a message across the cerebral centrum, where it is judged to be either a healthy or unhealthy influence. From the brain, this information is transmitted through the cerebral spine, then along nervous pathways (in this case, to the arms and hands and fingers), and is expressed in the muscular strength or weakness of the circle made by the person's fingers.

There exist unique and deep connections between the sensory and motor cortex of the brain and the hands. This allows the fingers to respond and reflect the judgment by the cerebral centrum. We could theoretically use any part of the body to gather this information, but due to this deep connection with the hands, we can get a more accurate response.

Another reason to use the fingers to carry out this test is because the finger muscles fatigue much less quickly than other muscle groups, allowing us to perform the test multiple times.

WHAT CAN WE DETERMINE FROM THIS TEST?

- normal and abnormal regions of the body
- the existence of internal substances, such as bacteria, virus, fungus, toxins, etc.
- the appropriateness of various Chinese medicinal herbs and formulas, supplements, foods, drinks, etc. for the individual's body

PREPARATION FOR THE VEM TEST:

- All electronic devices, such as a television, a microwave oven, infrared, ultrasound, etc. must be turned off. We make an exception for lighting in the room.
- The examiner as well as the patient must remove wrist watch, necklace, ring, glasses, the change in a pocket, a key, cell phone, medicine, etc. Anything that has an electromagnetic

field must be removed from the body before the test. It is not enough for the phone to be turned off, it must be removed from the body completely.
- Polarity Test:
  - Valid: The patient makes a closed circle with their fingers. Their other hand is placed palm-down on the forehead, then checked again palm-up. If the circle is able to be broken on one and not the other, then the case is valid for VEM test.

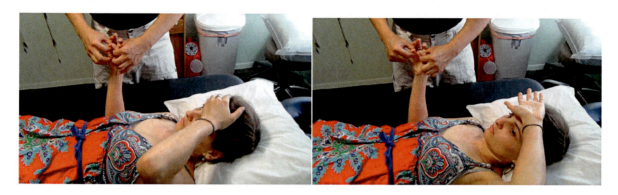

  - Invalid: If the circle is unable or able to be broken both ways, palm-up and palm-down, then the test is un-usable for VEM test.
    - Occasionally, when the patient is dehydrated the Polarity Test comes up as invalid. I suggest that the patient drink some water and to wait a few minutes, then repeat the test.
- Cervical vertebrae test: it is used to test validity of the test,
  - The circle is tested and should be closed even when the neck is turned left, right, up or down. If the circle opens, the patient is not a candidate for the VEM test.

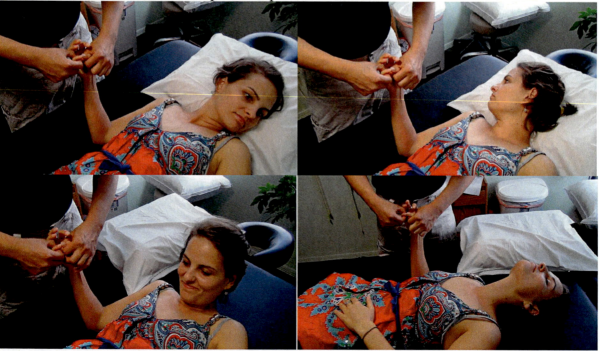

- In the case of a test being invalid, a research associate or a third party are needed. I will explain the way later.
- The test can be done in standing, sitting, or supine position.
- The patient's hands must be at least 8 inches away from the body.
- I recommend that the patient is not on carpet, due to static electricity.

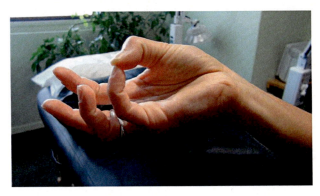

Ask the patient to connect the right thumb and small finger, making a circle.

The examiner will grasp the patient's thumb by connecting the thumb and index finger. With the other hand, the examiner will grasp the patient's small finger by connecting the thumb and index finger. In this way the examiner will be positioned to pull apart the circle made by the patient with his or her own hands.

The examiner asks the patient to hold their fingers gently together. Then he will lightly pull in opposite directions to pull the fingers apart.

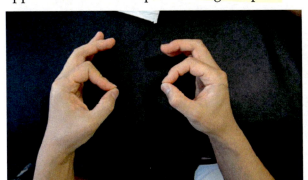
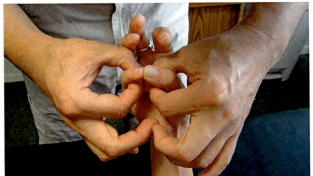

The patient concentrates on just lightly maintaining contact with the two fingers. It is important that the patient does not engage the muscles strongly in order to create the circle.

It is important to teach the patient what level of strength is necessary to maintain their fingers together. The examiner will test the circle with one ring. If the patient's fingers open with this pressure, they are holding too lightly. The ideal strength of the circle should be that the examiner is not able to open the patient's circle with their own thumb-index finger circle, but rather with the circle created by the thumb, index and middle fingers.

HOW TO INTERPRET RESULTS

"Level 0" is how I describe the test results when I am able to open the patient's fingers easily with just my own thumb-index finger circle.

If I am unable to open their circle with just my thumb and index finger, but need to use the thumb, index, and middle fingers, I define this as "base finger" or "level 1." If the addition of the ring finger is necessary to open the patient's circle, this is categorized as "level 2." If I must add the small finger as well, this is "level 3." Finally, if I am unable to open their circle with all four fingers I call this a "level 4." This is the maximum.

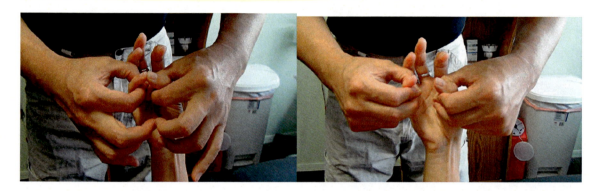

LEVEL 0   LEVEL 1

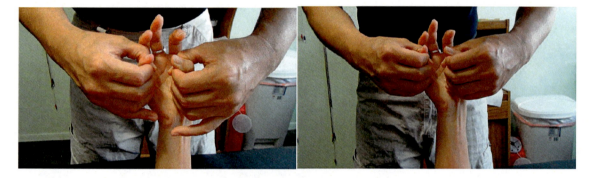

LEVEL 2   LEVEL 3

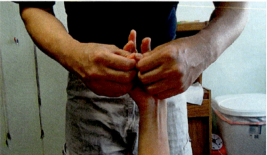

LEVEL 4

This system is very helpful in finding the appropriate supplement, herbal formula, and dosage. If I would like to test various internal organs of the patient, for example thymus, liver, pancreas, stomach, etc. I lightly and briefly make contact with that point with the tip of my thumb, after which I perform the VEM test on the patient's circle.

PERFORMING THE VEM TEST WITH THE HELP OF AN ASSISTANT

The test is performed in essentially the same way, the only difference being that an assistant uses his/her hand as the test subject rather than directly with the patient. Any metal stick, about 2mm in diameter and 8 inches in length, is appropriate to carry out this test. The stick is held at the top with the left hand and placed lightly on the appropriate point on the body of the patient. The assistant's right hand will form the circle between the index finger and thumb.

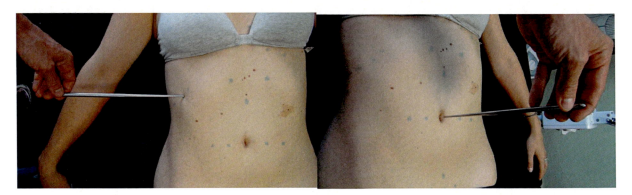

Testing the Liver   Testing the Small Intestine

This is my preferred method of doing the VEM test for two reasons: because it is quicker and more accurate. Quicker because I can skip the initial testing necessary to be done on the patient to determine their base-line strength. I believe that our thoughts can affect the test results, and having an assistant can help protect from the influence of my own preconceptions and impressions. Moreover, the use of an assistant allows us to perform the test when it is inconvenient to test the patient directly – i.e. on babies/children, on person's with missing fingers/limbs, patients with local injuries on the hands or fingers, patients with severe arthritis, etc.

IMPORTANCE OF THE THYMUS

Although the test can be performed on any part of the body, I give the most importance to the thymus. Only the Thymus responds in the opposite way as the other points on the body – it should result in a "level 0". In other words, the indication for a healthy Thymus is for the fingers to be open, whereas elsewhere on the body the person's circle should stay closed with the test. For this reason, the Thymus test is absolutely crucial in this system in order to be able to differentiate. Therefore, please keep in mind that the Thymus and other organ points should produce opposite results – if not, we need to go back and test the person with the Polarity Test, check the assistant, or check the Base Finger of the patient.

This can help prevent us from misinterpreting the test results.

The thymus gland is an endocrine organ which circulates T-lymphocytes (which is a lympholeukocyte) throughout the entire body, thus playing a very important role in the immune system. I believe that this very important gland acts as a sensor in the body, indicating whether the body is in balance or not.

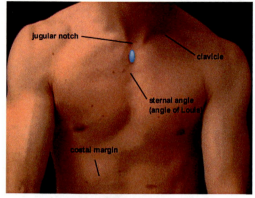

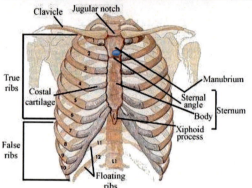

Therefore when selecting appropriate herbal medicine, supplements, and dosage, I first check for the thymus point to result in a Level 0 (fingers open), and the stomach, small intestine, and any other problematic area to result in a Level 4. (I check the stomach and small intestine because they are so critical in absorption – if their digestive system can't absorb the supplement we give, what is the use in prescribing it?) If there is trouble in the digestive system, I often make adjustments in dosage or form – i.e. liquid vs. capsules, etc.

The minimum results for the VEM to indicate positive for a person is Level 0 for the thymus point and at least Level 1 for the other organs. This is how we compare different products – the best choice is to get Level 4 on all test points along with the thymus open. But if it is not possible to get Level 4, perhaps we can be happy with Level 3. Testing supplements and food are different – for supplements I tend to want higher levels and for food I can be happy with just level 1 or 2. When comparing herbs or products, I tend to rank them – Level 4 is the most compatible or appropriate, and down to Level 1. This means that Level 1 is still compatible or appropriate for the person, but not as strong as Level 4. The only exception is the thymus, where level 0 is still indicative of a healthy interaction.

PRACTICALITY IN THE CLINIC

This is a simple way to perform a muscle test – we do not have to test all organs and points. We can perform a quick and accurate test with just these few points.

One interesting phenomenon of this test is that it is possible to find a substance that ranks as a Level 4, which would suggest that it is highly suitable for the person. However, if after testing this substance you find something else that is even more appropriate, the rank of the initial substance may change. An example: We may test a person for the formula Xiao Chai Hu Tang and get Level 4 results from the muscle testing. After the test, we reconsider the person's case and are curious about a different formula, Da Chai Hu Tang. When we test the latter, we find that it also gives us a Level 4 result. We go back and test Xiao Chai Hu Tang and find that it no longer gives us a Level 4 results, but rather a Level 3 or 2 result on different organs. This is quite mysterious. Perhaps we can say that the brain is somehow able to pick up on the subtle energy from the substance and is able to reconsider now that it has been exposed to the new information.

The test results depend very much on the examiner – which means that the breadth of knowledge and experience of the practitioner can allow for a better prescription for the patient, and the healing can progress much faster. You can't test something if you don't know about it or carry it in your pharmacy!

NOTE: It is very important because we need to continuously adjust our prescription as the treatment progresses – once certain symptoms improve we can discontinue the formula and/or make adjustments. It is not necessary to blindly prescribe formulas for extended periods of time, even if the person appears to have a chronic condition.

A SIMPLE CASE STUDY:

You have done the intake and palpation for a patient and believe that they are a candidate for a Liver *qi* stagnation formula. You have many formulas to choose from, how do you know which?

Kan Traditional: Free and Easy Wanderer (Xiao Yao San)

Kan Herbals: Relaxed Wanderer

Golden Flower: Bupleurum and Tang Kuei Formula

They are all, theoretically, the same formula. They should all work the same. In my experience, this is not true. Also if you look in the guidebooks, the indications are slightly different:

Bupleurum and Tang Kuei Formula: Typical Liver *qi* stagnation symptoms, also includes constipation as key indication

Relaxed wanderer: Liver *qi* stagnation symptoms but also with and loose stool.

Free and Easy Wanderer: Doesn't specify either loose stool or constipation.

Sometimes you carry the correct patent for the patient, but not all clinicians carry several brands of the same formula. What do you do if the patent doesn't work? Do you keep going until it does? The VEM test can help us figure out if it is working, the proper dosage, and whether or not a different patent of the same name can work better.

LOCATION OF TEST POINTS

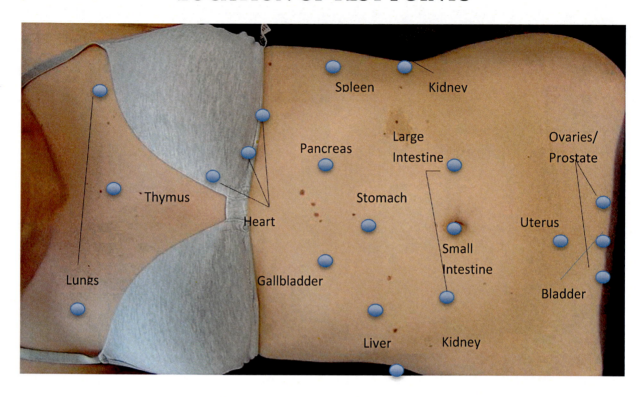

Stomach: Ren 11, 12 and 13. You should check all three points.

Small Intestine: Ren 8

Liver: Check the intercostal space of ribs 7, 8 and 9 (these correspond to Lr 14 and GB 24 and in between)

Kidney: Supine you can check GB 25. Prone you check BL 52

Large Intestine: Front-mu, ST 25 and Sp 15

Spleen: Along the left flank between the 7, 8 and 9 ribs

Pancreas: At the level of Ren 15, immediately to the left, at the edge of the ribcage

Gallbladder: At the level of Ren 15, immediately to the right, at the edge of the ribcage.

Lung: Lu 1

Heart: four points: Kd 22- Kd 24 and ST 18, all on the left side

Bladder: Check both Ren 2 and Ren 3

Uterus: Between Ren 3-4

Prostate/Ovaries: ST 30 – ST 29

Thymus: at the level of the sternal angle (angle of Louis). The point is in the center of the sternum. I find this point by gently sliding my finger down from the sternal notch until my finger stops at the slightly elevate angle.

CONCLUSION

The final decision is yours. You must choose based on diagnosis, experience, symptoms, and sense of what will be more cohesive for the patient.

It is a blend of intuition and intellect. It is normal for different practitioners to get different results.

Since incorporating this test into my practice, I achieved much quicker results, longer lasting changes, and more responsive and rapid ways of making changes.

The VEM test is a tool. Used appropriately it can be of tremendous benefit in your clinic.

HERBAL PRESCRIPTION PROCESS

In order to arrive at a correct herbal prescription, I rely on Traditional Chinese Medicine theory for differentiation of patterns. I begin with the Four observations, which leads me to differentiation based on Zang-Fu and Eight Principles, as well as Western disease diagnosis.

These theories frame my selection of two to four or five formulas that address both their chief complaint as well as underlying root/constitutional issues. I do not use the traditional diagnosis methods tongue and pulse diagnosis. Rather, I use the VEM test to determine the most suitable formula. I also consider nutritional supplements such as vitamins/minerals and western herbs along with my Chinese herbal formula prescription.

Typically I don't prescribe herbs on a patient's first visit. If by their second or third visit their condition hasn't changed much, or if the patient can't come often, I start thinking about combining Chinese herbs.

I prescribe the smallest possible quantity of herbal formula. I also prescribe only 1-2 weeks until next appointment so that we can determine if the formula is truly suitable and their chief complaint actually improves. By prescribing for a short period, this allows me to adjust formula and dosage if necessary. For chronic conditions, I recommend two pills, twice a day. In acute cases I prescribe two pills, three times per day, always on an empty stomach. I start with Golden Flower or Kan Herbals because their recommended dose is already 2 pills at a time. Other brands often suggest a higher dosage, and I try to keep my fees as low as possible for my patients and try to use the minimum dosage necessary to make a change.

I typically ask the patient to allow three treatments to determine if there is improvement in their chief complaint. The more frequently they can come, the better chance for improvement we will have, so this is why it is important to keep my fees as low as possible.

If after a taking herbs for a few weeks the patient's condition has improved and the formula seems to be working, I may continue with the prescription or use the VEM test to determine if I need to reduce the dosage. If the condition is not improving, or only slightly so, I use the VEM test to determine whether another formula is necessary, an additional formula should be combined to their prescription, or an adjustment is needed in the dosage.

I don't necessarily keep the patient on the initial formula once their chief complaint has improved or resolved. I consider adding a formula to address the root cause of their problems to combine with the formula they are currently taking for their symptoms. I often consider formulas from Health Concerns and Seven Forests as part of this combination.

When combining formulas, the additional formula is prescribed at chronic case: 2 pills, twice a day acute: 2 pills, three times per day. This means that each formula is taken at a dosage of 2 pills 2x/day for chronic situations or 2 pills 3x/day for acute and may mean that the patient is taking 4 or 6 pills total (2 or 3 respectively from each formula). This is prescribed for two weeks at a time.

Each dosage should be less than 4 tablets or capsules. I never prescribe more than two kinds of Chinese herbal patent medicines. However, in addition to the two herbal formulas I may include enzymes, probiotics, fiber, vitamins, minerals (nutritional supplements).

With Chinese herbs, taking more doesn't necessarily produce a better result. If the appropriate formula is prescribed, you should see improvement after just one or two weeks. This is how the VEM test can really aid us in selecting the correct formula for a condition. I learned in school that a person should take a formula for at least a couple months before seeing results. In my experience, if the correct formula and dosage are chosen, at the very least you should see improvement.

I use the following charts to be guided to the appropriate formula(s) and the VEM test to help me make a decision. I have a minimalist approach to herbal prescription. This is very similar to my acupuncture approach.

A CLINICAL MANUAL OF PRACTICAL ORIENTAL MEDICINE

GENERAL TEMPLATE FOR HERBAL PRESCRIPTION

PAIN IN UPPER BODY

HEADACHE/SINUS AND UPPER LIMBS (NECK/SHOULDER AND ELBOW, WRIST, JOINTS)

GOLDEN FLOWER	KAN	HEALTH CONCERNS	SEVEN FOREST	EVERGREEN
<ul><li>Head Relief</li><li>Blood Palace</li><li>Bupleurum Tang Kuei</li><li>Free and Easy Wanderer Plus</li><li>Bupleurum D</li><li>Bupleurum and Cinnamon</li><li>Gastrodia and Uncaria</li></ul>	<ul><li>Subdue Head Wind</li><li>Free and Easy Wanderer</li><li>Bupleurum Smoothing Liver</li><li>Meridian Comfort</li><li>Graceful Branches</li><li>Bi Yan Pian</li><li>Calm Dragon</li></ul>	<ul><li>Head-Q</li><li>Ease 2</li><li>Ease Plus</li><li>Coptis Purge Fire</li><li>Channel Flow</li><li>Gastrodia Relieve Wind</li><li>Mobility 3</li><li>SP2M</li></ul>	<ul><li>Angelica 14</li><li>Bupleurum 12</li><li>Chrysanthemum 9</li><li>Cnidium 9</li><li>Gastrodia 9</li><li>Gentiana 12</li><li>Pueraria 10</li><li>Pueralex</li><li>Upper Palace</li></ul>	<ul><li>Neck & Shoulder (Acute)</li><li>Neck & Shoulder (Chronic)</li><li>Herbal Analgesic</li><li>Migratrol</li><li>Corydalin</li><li>Arm Support</li></ul>

PAIN IN LOWER BODY

LOW BACK/HIP AS WELL AS LOWER LIMBS (KNEE/ANKLE/FEET)

GOLDEN FLOWER	KAN	HEALTH CONCERNS	SEVEN FOREST	EVERGREEN
<ul><li>Course and Quicken</li><li>Du Huo and Loranthus</li><li>Chase Wind Penetrate Bone</li><li>Restorative</li><li>Bone and Sinew</li><li>Tang Kuei and Peony</li><li>Essential Yang</li><li>Rehmannia Six</li><li>True Yin</li><li>Corydalis</li><li>Two Immortals</li></ul>	<ul><li>Angelic ad Eucommia Support</li><li>Clear Channel</li><li>Invigorate the Collaterals</li><li>Meridian Comfort</li><li>Meridian Passage</li><li>Benefit Hip and Knee</li><li>Two Immortals</li><li>Female Comfort</li></ul>	<ul><li>Mobility 2</li><li>Mobility 3</li><li>Backbone</li><li>AC-Q</li><li>Channel Flow</li><li>Three Immortals</li></ul>	<ul><li>Chiang Huo 13</li><li>Acanthopanax 10</li><li>Eucommia 18</li><li>Liquidamber 15</li><li>Corydalis 5</li><li>Siler</li><li>Drynaria 12</li></ul>	<ul><li>Back Support (Chronic)</li><li>Back Support (HD)</li><li>Back Support (Acute)</li><li>Knee & Ankle (Chronic)</li><li>Knee & Ankle (Acute)</li><li>Flex (Spur)</li><li>Herbal Analgesic</li></ul>

*Please consult the clinical handbook offered by each company to seek suggestions for combining formulas. Evergreen Herbs are prescribed either as a single formula at their recommended dosage of 3-4 pills per dose, or when combining, I prescribe only 2 pills per dose.

HEAT THERAPY IN TREATMENT

The use of heat as part of therapy cannot be underestimated. Aside from Neijing theory which encourages us to fear cold and embrace warmth, years of clinical experience have supported that suggestion. Most patients present with cold somewhere on the body, very typically cold feet. Almost all patients benefit from applying warmth at the neck, abdomen, lower back, or feet. This can happen during treatment, with a TDP lamp or foot sauna, or post-treatment as homework for the patient with a heating pad or foot baths. Patients seem to improve much quicker when they are also doing heat therapy at home concurrently with the acupuncture and herbal treatments. Something as simple as 15 minutes of heating pad per night before bed on the neck can go a long way not just for neck and shoulder tension, but to healing internal disorders as well.

Moxa, while a cornerstone of most acupuncturists' practice, is rarely used in this system. Many Japanese practitioners use dozens of tiny, "rice-grain" sized moxa stimulations at the point of insertion in order to potentiate the effects of the point. In clinical practice, working alone, I rarely have time to perform such laborious procedures, so my style has developed accordingly. Occasionally the use of smokeless incense or Moxsafe needle moxa will be applied at points, but again, this is rare. More often than not, the foot sauna and TDP lamps take the place of moxa. You are encouraged to develop your practice according to your own experience and interests. If you love moxa, do it!

POST-ACUPUNCTURE TREATMENT FINE-TUNING AND CARE

As mentioned before, one of the most important aspects of this system is patient satisfaction. Theory can go a long way, but until your patients see the benefits of our work, what is the point? This is why there is typically time dedicated at the end of the acupuncture session for "fine-tuning" or "touching-up".

This is the part of the treatment where you will ask the patient to re-evaluate their pain. The patient is to slowly get up from the table and move their head, neck, back, or whichever part that they felt pain before the treatment. If there is any lingering pain, stiffness, or discomfort, this final step is very important to do before they leave your clinic.

If their pain persists in the lower limbs, such as knee, ankle, foot or even hip, you will stimulate the HJL5 point which is ipsilateral to the pain. For this, the patient will stand and face the treatment table, placing palms down on the table allowing them to rest and slightly bend forward. You will insert the point while the patient is standing, and stimulate for a few seconds, and ask them to repeat the painful movement. Once their pain has diminished, you may remove the needles. RETENTION IS NOT NECESSARY AT THIS POINT. This point can also be used for any pain at the occiput.

If pain remains at the SI joint, the patient will stand in the same way against the table as you palpate and needle the most sensitive point around the SI 13 area. Needles are withdrawn after short stimulation and reduction of pain at the affected area.

For any other lingering spots of pain or tenderness, the Synthesis points are used in the same way described in that section. This time, however, they are not retained. They are stimulated briefly and removed. A press-needle may be left at the exact point where you placed the needle and you may request that the patient press on this point over the next few days to continue the treatment.

CASE STUDIES

The videos won't show detail about point locations, because the most important aspect of this kind of system has to do with the overall method, and each person will have a slightly different point location. I have included my patient notes below.

DVD DISC 1:

1. A.F. Female Age: 28

Chief Complaint: Migraine

Treatment: Yin Tang, outer ST 43, SJ 5, GB 26

Patient complains of headache at left temple, behind eye, and along eyebrow line, which started yesterday. She also says she feels very hot.

She reports that she is in the middle of her menstrual cycle, and also reports that she felt a bit nauseous the previous evening, and had trouble sleeping, making her feel irritable today.

Careful abdominal palpation reveals pain at bilateral ST 25 area, Ren 3, Ren 12, left Kd 16, and Liver area under ribcage.

Neck palpation shows Left Trapezius #1, 2 and 4 as well as SCM #2 and 3 to be tender. The left temple is also palpated and tenderness found at Tai Yang, ST 2, Yu Yao, and BL 2.

After palpation, the VEM test is performed. This is a good example of showing how I test the patient first to see if the VEM test will be valid. This is done by checking her with the palm up and down on her forehead. Because she felt hot and is in the middle of her cycle, I considered it to potentially be a hormonal condition. My first thought was a more traditional formula Chai Hu Shu Gan Wan, but I needed to do the VEM test to be sure. I first checked the Women's Balance formula at the Thymus point, and find it to be open, which is a good sign, so I continue with the other points at the Stomach and Small Intestine and find them to be closed, which is also a positive sign. For now, this seems to be a good choice for her, but I decide to try another formula for her, which is Kan's Bupleurum Soothing Liver Formula. I find it to close the Thymus point, which is an immediate sign that the formula is not appropriate for her. I tested Women's Balance formula again, just to be sure, and it seems to be a very good choice. I next tried Headache Cure formula to compare it with Women's Balance, and it seemed that Women's Balance ended up being the strongest choice. 3 pills TID was her prescription.

Acupuncture treatment begins with the Yin Tang point, because Ren 12, Ren 3 and Kd 16 were found to be tender upon palpation. The right ST 25 and left ST 27 were left over after the first needle. Because she was tender at BL 2 and Yu Yao on the left, I couldn't use the essential points to release her abdomen. I chose outer ST 43 based on palpation between that and ST 43. I chose this point because she really didn't show any Spleen symptoms. This seemed to relieve the tenderness along the Trapezius as well as BL 2, Yu Yao, Tai Yang and ST 2. SCM #2 was still tender, so I chose left SJ 5 at a tender location for the next treatment point. This relieved the remaining tenderness at the left SCM #2. At this point she reported that her migraine had improved but still painful behind the eye, especially when looking to the side. The next point I chose was GB 26 for the pain behind the eye. I chose this point from clinical experience, as it seems to work better for me than GB 41 for pain behind the eye.

Needles were left for 20 minutes.

After the treatment, she was asked to sit up and check to see if any pain remained. Mostly her headache was gone, but still there was some pain left over at BL 1 area. BL 62 was needled at the most tender spot while she was sitting in order to reduce the remaining pain at BL 1.

2. R.P. Female Age: 54

Chief Complaint: heartburn, neck shoulder tension, upset stomach after eating, arch of the foot pain bilaterally at Kd 2 area.

Treatment: Yin Tang, BL 2, Kd 6

I first need to determine whether she is responsive to VEM test. For this the hand is placed palm down on the forehead, the ring is checked, and then the palm is placed palm-up on the forehead and then the ring checked again. If there is no difference between the two, then the patient is not going to be responsive to the VEM test. This may be due to dehydration, brain injury, neck injury, etc.

After deciding that she is responsive to the VEM test, I checked the Thymus point, and for her it is closed. The Stomach, Small Intestine, Large Intestine, Pancreas, Liver are all open VEM responses, meaning there is a problem.

I chose Shu Gan Wan from Health Concerns herbs. If the right herbs are chosen, the Thymus should be open, and the internal organs should be closed. I tried four strength levels, 1,2,3, and 4 to check for efficacy of the herbs. All organs responded with strength, suggesting that this is a good formula for her.

Just to be sure I checked Kan Herbs Shu Gan Wan, and Thymus point stayed closed. For the Stomach point, it stayed closed for strength test 1,2 and 3 but opened for #4.

Heartburn Essential from Pure Encapsulations was the third formula tested, to see if it should be combined with the Chinese herbs. This is an enzyme supplement, and I wanted to be sure if it would compliment her formula or not. I checked the Thymus, it is closed, Stomach opens at 3.

Lastly I combined the Heartburn Essentials with Health Concerns Shu Gan Wan, and Thymus didn't open, and Stomach opened at 3. This means that it made things weaker, so it meant that Heartburn Essential wasn't necessary this time.

I prescribed Health Concerns Shu Gan Wan, 2 pills, 3x/day.

Abdominal Palpation: ST 25 and ST 27 on left are tender, Ren7, right ST 27, Ren 12, Ren 13, Ren14 Pancreas reflection area, Gall Bladder reflection area, Liver reflection area,

Neck Palpation: Left trapezius: #2, #3,and # 4 and SCM #2 and # 3

Right Trapezius: #2 and # 3, SCM #2, #3

Treatment: Yin Tang, bilateral BL 2 because all three front zones showed tenderness. Abdomen cleared completely with these points. Neck still sore at Trap #2, and left at right instep. Kd 6 was selected to address the foot pain. With this needle the foot pain resolved and the neck improved as well, so no further needles were necessary.

3. J.P. Male Age: 80

Chief Complaint: Right wrist, diagnosis of carpal tunnel syndrome.

This is his second visit in the clinic, first treatment was last week. History of right sided inguinal hernia and surgery on neck for clogged arteries. Some blockage still exists. Chief complaint is hand pain.

Treatment: Right BL 2, Right Lr 3, Right GB 41

Begins with palpation of hand. Palpation revealed tenderness at the Lung and Large Intestine channels on the hand – Lu 9, Lu 10, LI 5. Afterwards, careful palpation of the neck zones, with tenderness at Trapezius # 2 and #3, and SCM # 2, #3, and #4 (which is brachial plexus area).

Stomach palpation follows, with tenderness at Liver zone – both under the ribs and at the right groin/ASIS area where he had scar tissue from inguinal hernia surgery.

RELEVANT PALPATION: Chief complaint is most important. I palpate areas that I feel are connected or are relevant areas to his complaint. If I were to palpate the whole body surely I would find tenderness everywhere and this can divert my treatment from being so focused. Keep your acupuncture message simple while still considering the whole body. If on the following treatment I don't find much improvement, I might search elsewhere for more of a source or deeper root to this problem. In his case, his symptoms resolved quite quickly, within a few treatments.

Findings: From a zone perspective, symptoms show up on right side, especially right side of neck, right hand, Liver, right groin, etc. This leads me to choose BL 2 on the right as my Essential point treatment. After needling BL 2, re-check areas for tenderness, and found that Trap #2 and SCM still tender. Lr 3 is chosen to try to release more of the neck. In this case, the neck released at the right side of C3 vertebrae and along the SCM, but remained at the ASIS. GB 41/42 was palpated, and 42 was chosen because it was more tender. This released the remaining tenderness at the ASIS.

Finally, the wrist was re-palpated for tenderness and was found to not be tender at all. This is the end of treatment.

This is a clear case of how internal organ involvement as well as neck tension can manifest as pain in the hand.

4. T.G. Female Age: 29

Chief Complaint: Neck pain on left, radiating into shoulder blades. Low back pain on right side

Treatment: Du 17, BL 9, SJ 5

Patient is asked to show movements that cause pain.

The VEM test is performed with the help of an assistant. I mark the Thymus, Ren 12 (ST) and Ren 8 (SI). Thymus point was closed, and the Stomach and Small Intestine points were open. I compared three formulas – Meridian Passage, Invigorate the Collaterals, and Meridian Comfort, all from Kan – to check which would be most appropriate. Since The first two formulas didn't cause the Thymus point to be open, I decided they were not appropriate. Since Meridian Comfort successfully caused the Thymus point to be open I continued with the test on the Stomach and Small Intestine points over Ren 12 and 8 respectively. It caused both points to be closed, which is a positive sign for those points, so I chose Meridian Comfort as my herbal prescription to accompany the acupuncture treatment.

Since most of her pain is on her back, the patient was asked to lay prone and her spine, shoulders and low back were palpated for tenderness and marked with a highlighter. Tender spots were found all along the spine as well as the around the sacrum and at the SI joint. The Bladder channel was also checked and marked for tenderness

Acupuncture treatment begins at Du 17 and the spine is again palpated. Since there was a significant reduction in tenderness all along the spine and shoulders Du 17 was not stimulated again.

Some tenderness remained at the outer Bladder channel line starting at the level of T7 to L2 on the right side. BL 9 on the right was needled, which was sufficient to eliminate any remaining tenderness along the Bladder channel. The neck was then palpated again for tenderness, and some was found bilaterally along the SCM. SJ 5 was needled and gently vibrated for a few seconds to release these tender zones.

Needles were left for 25 minutes and heat was applied to the upper and lower back.

Herbs: meridian comfort from Kan 2 pills 2x/day

5. G.R. Female Age: 67

Chief complaint: right sciatica pain

Treatment: Du 17, HJL5, GB 25

Pain is along spine with a shooting pain down right thigh and leg.

Patient is asked to lie prone for palpation along back and right hip and leg. Tender spots are carefully marked along the Gall Bladder channel on the hip – including the joint area and piriformis muscle. Many points along the sacrum were found to be tender as well. The lumbar spine was palpated, with tenderness found at L4-L5, and the Bladder channel seemed to be fairly pain free. The right SI joint was also very tender. The IT band was palpated all the way down the Gall Bladder channel to the knee, and marked where tender.

Treatment begins with needling Du 17, and the low back and hip are palpated again. Tenderness remains at the spine at L4-L5 so the point is removed and a new location is found and Du 17 is needled again in a slightly different location. Now, points are palpated there is significant reduction in pain although not completely, so the needle is gently vibrated for a few more seconds, which helps reduce the tenderness along the spine and hip even more. The SI joint and hip are less tender as well, with just a few remaining tender spots left at the GB channel along the thigh. The right Huatuo Jiaji of L5 is needled and gently stimulated. This reduces the tenderness along the Gall Bladder channel and lateral thigh. GB 25 is needled at a tight, tender spot and gently vibrated as a support point for the treatment.

Needles were retained for 20 minutes with heat lamp at the low back.

After the treatment patient was asked to stand up slowly from the treatment table and move around, and she reported that she felt no pain or restriction in movement, so no touch-ups were necessary.

6. T.L. Female Age: 35

Chief complaint: left inner-knee pain, left sciatic pain

Treatment: Du 17, left HJL5, left Lr 3, left Kd 6

Patient is questioned about history and asked to demonstrate positions or movement that cause pain. Pain is at left SI joint/hip/sciatic as well.

VEM test done for herbal formula: Abdomen and local inner-knee area were checked as well as Thymus.

Two formulas, both from Evergreen Herbs, were prescribed at 2 pills TID: Knee & Ankle (Chronic) and Back Support (HD). Tests were done for the individual formulas, then tested again with both formulas in her hand. Thymus point remained open with these formulas, so it was deemed appropriate.

These herbs were selected because she had come in one month before with a similar condition, and she said that it really helped. She requested that she be prescribed more herbs, so the VEM test was done in order to determine if the formulas were still appropriate.

Inner knee was palpated and tender area marked with the highlighter. Sp 9, Lr 8, and Kd 10 found tender. Abdomen palpated, groin and left ASIS were the only tender area. She was asked to lay on her side in order to palpate the low back and left hip where she complained of "sciatic" pain. Tenderness at L3-L5 and S1, as well as along sacrum and piriformis muscle (GB 30, 29, 28, Japanese GB 27).

She is lying on her side for treatment, Du 17 needled first because found pain along spine and Jiaji. Pain left at GB 29. Left Jiaji of L5 was needled because it is indicated for tenderness/pain at regions of Gall Bladder and Bladder channels below L5, and her chief complaint is knee pain of that side, so this point has multiple reasons for use.

Needles left in for 15 minutes while side-lying with a heat lamp on low back area.

Afterwards she was asked to lay supine, and knee palpated again, with points found tender at Liver and Kidney meridians. Groin is better, as well as ASIS.

Lr 3 is chosen and knee re-palpated. Kd 6 then selected for remaining pain along Kideny channel. Needles are not retained.

After she is asked to stand and walk around. Since no pain remaining in hip or knee there are no post-treatment needles necessary.

7. P.L. Female Age: 49

Chief Complaint: Left-sided TMJ

Treatment: BL 2, Tai Yang, Sp 4, SJ 5, GB 26, ST 43

Palpation begins at the jaw, along Stomach and Small Intestine channels, and marked with a non-toxic highlighter. In this case, the patient is asked to find the spots herself and then I mark them. Patient reports that the TMJ began the previous morning. This is the third time she has had severe TMJ pain.

After palpation the patient was asked to demonstrate how much she could open and close her jaw.

The neck is then carefully palpated along the left side and found to be tender all along Trapezius and SCM zones.

Abdomen is palpated, and found to be tender at the Spleen Zone as well as left ST 25 –Sp 15 area.

Treatment begins with BL 2 on the left as well as the left Tai Yang point. After, the left Sp 4 is needled and gently vibrated.

Abdomen is re-palpated and Spleen Zone is still tender, as well as some tenderness at the left C3. Jaw is still painful along Stomach channel.

SJ 5 is needled at a tender spot in order to address the remaining tenderness at the SJ 21 area. GB 26 is needled at a tender spot because the jaw pain is within the GB 26 zone. Patient is asked to try to open her jaw now, and point to where pain lingers. ST 43 is checked again and the pain is significantly reduced.

Needles are retained for 30 minutes, heat lamp was applied to the jaw area. After the needles were removed, the patient was asked to sit up and re-evaluate the jaw pain. Some tenderness remained along the San Jiao channel, and SJ 5 was needled at a tender spot and the jaw was checked again. The needle was removed after about one minute and a press needle was left in place at SJ 5.

8. G.K. Male Age: 68

Chief Complaint: Neck, Low back, IT band pain

Treatment: Du 17, SJ 5, GB 26, Kd 6, BL 62

First, the spine is palpated from neck to sacrum, marking tender points along the way. Next the BL channel is palpated and tender areas marked. The right IT band is palpated and marked where the patient says there is numbness.

Du 17 is selected first because of so much tenderness along the spine. After insertion and gentle vibrations at the needle, the spine is palpated again. There is a significant reduction all along the spine. The Bladder channel along the neck and back are also palpated, and it seems that this time Du 17 alone was enough to reduce tenderness along those areas as well. Some pain remains at the left and right side of the neck at the SCM muscles and marked with a different color. SJ 5 is needled bilaterally for this issue.

The IT band is palpated again, and the patient reports that there is improvement in the numbness in the area with a little tenderness along the GB 31-32 area. GB 26 on the right is needled at the most tender spot. A little gentle stimulation is needed to fully release the tenderness along the IT band.

Kd 6 and BL 62 were palpated bilaterally for tenderness. Kd 6 on the left was found to relieve the left low back tenderness, and BL 62 on the right was the point which relieved the remaining tenderness at the right low back.

Needles are retained for 25 minutes, and a heat lamp is placed over upper and lower back.

DVD DISC 2:

9. D.D. Female Age: 45

Chief Complaint: low back pain and left shoulder pain.

Treatment: Du 17, right BL 9, left GB 12, left SI 3

Palpation begins with the low back. Even though her chief complaint is on the right side, palpation of the left low back and hip is also done. Du channel points and BL 50 – 52 and Yao Yan point is tender, and BL 25 and BL 26. Notice how the sacrum is palpated. Left shoulder is also palpated carefully around the shoulder blade and down the arm. Small Intestine and San Jiao channels are tender along upper arm. Upper thoracic vertebrae are tender. SCM muscle is tender on the left side.

Du 17 needled first, upward with the channel, then the back rechecked.

There are points at the right L4 vertebrae that are tender, as well as bilateral sacrum points, close to GB 30.

Du 17 stimulated slightly again, and BL 9 on right needled to address lingering issues at lower back. This released all remaining tender spots at the low back.

Left shoulder checked.

GB12 needled at most tender spot.

Left over pain at shoulder is along Small Intestine channel, so SI 3-4 area is palpated and needled at the most tender spot. This relieved the remaining pain at the posterior shoulder.

10. G.L. Female Age: 48

Chief Complain: acute low back pain

Treatment: Du 17, BL 9, BL 62, GB 25

Patient arrived with acute low back pain, saying that it was very painful when sitting and bending over. I began with palpation of her back of tender spots, starting with the spine, and carefully marking each spot with a non-toxic highlighter. Although she came in with the complaint of "low-back pain," palpation revealed that it was more her mid-back that was more sensitive. The SI joint and hips were also tender to palpation. Acupuncture treatment began with Du 17 to address the tenderness along the spine. Once needled, her back was re-palpated and checked for improvement. I found that I could press harder without causing pain, and the improvement applied not only to her spine but also to the rest of her back. This is a good example of how one Essential point can influence beyond its zone, and why careful placement of the needle is useful in really "clearing the field" to see what needs to happen next.

BL 23 and 53 as well as Lumbar Eyes were still tender on the left, so BL 9 on the left was needled. This relieved the tenderness at those spots. A few tender areas were left around the sacrum on her left side.

Given that this is an acute situation, and that tenderness remained in the BL zone, I chose to palpate for a tender spot at her left BL 62, and when needled it relieved the tenderness at all remaining spots.

To support the treatment I added GB 25 bilaterally. After the treatment she felt no pain, so no fine-tuning was necessary.

11. A.F. Female Age: 28

Chief Complain: Low back pain on right side, and temporal headache and jaw pain

Treatment: Du 17, Du 14, SJ 5

Palpation began with the patient in lateral-recumbent position. I started with the hip and low back area before I thoroughly checked the neck, temple and jaw. Of course, I marked all tender spots with a highlighter.

Tenderness was found at the right hip and along the spine at the mid and low-back, as well as GB 20 area, SCM, temple (along SJ and GB channels), and jaw.

Treatment began with Du 17 to address the tenderness found along the spine in the neck and low back. Tenderness still remained at the right SI joint but not along the spine, so I gently vibrated the needle again at Du 17. Because pain was still found at the L5-S1 area, I needled Du 14 as a support point. This was effective in reducing the remaining tenderness at the low back as well as the hip.

After the low-back was addressed, I moved on to check the neck again. Tenderness was still found at SCM #2, so I needled SJ 5 at the most tender location. This was effective in reducing the tenderness at the SCM, temple and jaw.

Because her feet were cold, I decided to offer the foot sauna.

After 20 minutes, needles were removed and she was asked to reevaluate her pain in the neck and jaw, as well as the low back. The neck and jaw had improved greatly. Her low back was still a bit "sore" at the SI joint, so I decided to add SI 13 on the right. After a 30 seconds the needle was removed, and she reported that her pain had improved.

12. M.G. Female Age: 59

Chief Complaint: shoulder/arm pain, numbness in wrist at LI 5 area

Treatment: BL 2, Tai Yang, Lr 3, LI 4

Begins with careful palpation. Tenderness found along Large Intestine and Lung channels all the way down to wrist

Then careful palpation of the neck, especially on the affected side

All areas of the Trapezius and SCM muscles are tender. Abdominal palpation reveals Liver zones, Brachial plexus is among the tender areas

Abdomen – Liver area, Spleen area, navel

BL 2 is needled to address Liver zone issues, and Tai Yang needled to address right arm issues. Neck still tender all over, Tai Yang removed and replaced, rechecked. San Jiao, Large Intestine, Small Intestine channels palpated for tenderness again. Lr 3 is added to address Liver zone.

Brachial plexus point tender, as well as wrist still numb/tender at LI 5 point, so LI 3-4 palpated and needled where most sensitive.

In this case it seems the Large Intestine channel is the most involved, and the brachial plexus point can be interpreted in this context as being related to the Large Intestine channel over the others.

Rechecked after acupuncture treatment, no further fine tuning necessary

13. P.S. Female Age: 63

Chief Complain: knee pain, bilateral

Treatment: BL 2, left Sp 4, right ST 43

Start with palpation of knees, and mark with non-toxic highlighter. Palpation of the groin is very relevant to the knee pain cases, as demonstrated in the video. In this case, the Spleen channels seem to be tender for her, as well as along the ASIS (GB channel).

Abdominal palpation reveals only ST 27 bilaterally is tender.

VEM test was done to check for herbs.

BL 2 is needled and then the abdomen and groin and knees are palpated again. This relieves tenderness in groin and most knee pain. Remaining tender spots are carefully checked and marked again with a different color. On the left knee, the remaining tender spots are mostly along the Spleen channel. On the right knee, the remaining tender areas are mostly along the Stomach channel. Treated with Sp 4 on the left, ST 43 on right.

Final touches are not necessary in this case, because there is no lingering pain.

14. E.M. Female Age: 54

Chief Complaint: Knee pain post-surgery

Treatment: BL 9, HJL5, Sp 4, BL 2, ST 43

Patient had knee replacement surgery on the right knee three weeks ago. She came for treatment for swelling, stiffness, pain and numbness at the scar. She had difficulty bending the knee. After surgery she had numbness at the bottom of the foot and in the calf. She also has a history of the right leg "being longer" than the other, making it difficult to walk without special shoes.

Treatment begins with careful palpation of the knee, and marking all areas which are numb or painful. The groin was also palpated and found to be tender along the Stomach and Spleen channels.

The abdomen was palpated and found to be tender at the right ASIS and inguinal ligament, especially on the right but a little on the left as well. After supine palpation, she was asked to roll over prone and have the knee, calf, and foot palpated for pain or numbness as well. Her thigh and back were palpated along the Bladder channels.

Treatment began supine, with BL 9 being the Essential point chosen because there was no tenderness along the spine or the Huatuo Jiaji points. The Bladder channel along the thigh and calf was palpated and found that most of the tender spots had been reduced. Some tenderness remained at the Kidney channel area. The HJL5 point was needled on the right side to address these tender areas remaining at the lower limb, which required a bit of gentle vibration at the needle in order to be completely effective. She still reported numbness at the lateral foot along the Bladder/Gall Bladder channels.

The front of the knee was palpated with the patient still prone, and the numbness and tenderness still remained at most areas, especially along the Spleen channel. Sp 4 was needled and it improved the numbness and tenderness at the knee.

The needles were retained for 20 minutes and then she was asked to turn over and have a supine treatment. The knee and foot were checked again for tenderness and numbness.

A needle was inserted at the right BL 2 point, and the knee was still found to be tender at the scar, the ankle at GB 40, but the ASIS/inguinal ligament tenderness had greatly improved. ST 43 was then palpated at two spots, and the traditional location of ST 43 was chosen because it was more tender than the outer ST 43 spot. Needles were retained for only a minute, and then withdrawn, after which she was asked to stand and walk around again. Even the leg length seemed to straighten out.

Please see the accompanying video for several follow-up treatments to see her progress over a few weeks.

14a. E.M. Female Age: 54

Chief Complaint: Knee pain post-surgery, follow-up one week later

Treatment: BL 9, HJL5, ST 43

Patient returned one week after previous treatment, saying that the knee is still very tender and "weird." She was asked to demonstrate which movements caused pain, and then palpation of the entire knee, front and back, began while she lay prone. All points around the knee were marked with a non-toxic highlighter. After knee palpation the back was also checked for tenderness, and all points marked.

BL 9 on the right was chosen first because nothing was tender along the spine, just along the BL channel and the right lower limb. All tender points were re-palpated for tenderness. Patient reported that all points along the BL channel were no longer tender. On the front of the knee, along the Sp and Lr channels, there were a few spots remaining. Because there was pain still at the knee, the right HJL5 point was needled. This seemed to improve the tenderness at the medial knee. Her knee was still feeling numb, but no longer painful. In places where it was previously numb, she reported that she could now feel pressure from palpation and a bit of tenderness on palpation. ST 43 and outer ST 43 were both palpated for tenderness, and ST 43 was needled because it was more tender upon palpation. This improved the numbness/pain that remained at the knee. A TDP lamp was left over her low back, and needles were retained for 20 minutes.

After the treatment she was asked to repeat the movements which cause her difficulty and pain to re-evaluate. The ankle and knee were both feeling much better, but still some lingered at the medial knee. The HJL5 point in the right was needled with the patient standing, gently vibrated with Synergetic Qi technique, and removed after a few seconds.

14b. E.M. Female Age: 54

Chief Complaint: Knee pain post-surgery, 2nd follow-up

Treatment: Du 17, BL 9, HJL5, outer ST 43

As with previous treatments, I start with palpation of the knee and mark all tender points. There seems to be less sensitivity in places where before there was pain, and more sensation at points where before there was only numbness. Careful palpation of the back follows.

Du 17 is needled first as it addresses the tenderness along the spine. After needling, tenderness remained at the right hip, so BL 9 on the right was needled.

Some pain was left at the right calf, so the right HJL5 was needled.

The patient felt pain still along the ST channel, so ST 43 was palpated for tenderness, and the outer ST 43 point was selected and needled. The point was gently vibrated for a few seconds in order to reduce the pain along the channel. Needles were retained for 20 minutes with TDP lamp placed over the low back and knee.

After the treatment she didn't report any pain, so no follow-up treatment was necessary.

CASES WITHOUT ACCOMPANYING VIDEO

15. J.A. Male Age: 54

Chief Complaint: Acute low back pain

Treatment: Du 17, BL 62

Pain began that morning, and patient had difficulty bending over or twisting from side to side.

The patient's back is palpated along the spine starting at the mid back and going down to the sacrum, marking tender spots. Bladder channel was also palpated and carefully marked. Dai Mai points along Gall Bladder channel were palpated, and GB 26 and 30 area were also tender. Because he had been coming to see me for chronic hamstring tightness and pain, I decided to palpate the right leg. When checking the Bladder and Gall Bladder channels along the thigh, several points were found to be tender as well.

Du 17 was needled first as the Essential point. After a few seconds of gentle vibration at the needle, the spine was checked again. Pain was reduced along the spine but remained at the Bladder channel on the right side in the BL 20-23 and 51-52 area as well as the left hip at GB 30 area.

The right Kd 6 and BL 62 points were palpated for tenderness. While doing acupressure at BL 62, I palpated the BL 51-52 area of the low back. Since it was significantly reduced, I chose to needle BL 62. Because this is an acute situation, and he has no Kidney deficiency symptoms it is more common to use BL 62 in these situations. BL 62 on the left was also needled to reduce pain and tenderness at the left hip and low back.

Needles were retained for 20 minutes with a heat lamp applied to the low back.

After the treatment the patient was asked to stand again and re-evaluate his low back pain. He still felt pain at the left low back and pins and needles across the low back. The left SI 13 was needled at a tender spot and gently vibrated for a few seconds to address the pain at the left SI joint area. The patient was then asked to move a little while the needle was in. Patient could then bend forward more, but the itchy, "ants biting" sensation remained along the spine. Du 14 was palpated for tenderness and needled at the most sensitive location and gently stimulated for a few seconds. The patient then reported that the itchy feeling resolved. The patient was then asked to bend again, and reported significant improvement in both pain and pins and needles feeling. The Du 14 and SI 13 points were then removed. Patient was counseled to continue treatment at home with heating pad at the low back.

16. E.L. Female Age: 67

Chief complaint: Right trapezius muscle pain, stiffness in right arm. Right low back pain

Treatment: Du 17, BL 9, SJ 5, SI 13 used as fine tuning after treatment.

Patient is first asked to show where she is feeling pain, and which movements cause more pain.

Next the VEM test is done to check which of her supplements are appropriate. Because she is taking so many supplements we want to see which are helpful and which may not be necessary. Those which do not open the Thymus point may not be necessary. Those which open the Thymus point and close the other organs are recommended. The dosage is based on how many pills are used while performing the test (i.e. if two pills are used, then that is the recommendation for dosage; in this way we can determine whether the dosage of a pill is appropriate.)

After checking her supplements, we check the Chinese herbs. I found that Bupleurum Tang Kuei from Golden Flower was the most appropriate for her condition, prescribed for two weeks, at 2 pills, 2x/day.

Next the abdomen is palpated. Tenderness is found at the left and right ST 27 area, Ren 4, 12-14 area, and around the navel at Kd 16 as well as along the right ribcage in the Liver zone.

The neck was palpated and found tender all along the Trapezius zone and SCM muscle on the right side, and the left SCM muscle.

Patient was then asked to lie prone on the table, and the shoulders and back were palpated and tender areas marked with a highlighter.

Treatment was given at Du 17 first, to address the tenderness along the spine at the neck and low back. Tenderness remained at L5 on the right side, so Du 17 was removed and needled again in a slightly different location. This slight change in point location helped release the tenderness along the spine and at L5 as well as along the Bladder channel and shoulders. The neck was still tender so BL 9 was needled, which didn't completely resolve the tenderness at the SCM muscle, just at the BL 10 area. SJ 5 on the right was then needled to address the right-sided SCM tenderness.

After the treatment, the patient was asked to stand. She still felt pain at the right side of neck and low back, so some additional needling was necessary. SJ 5 on the right was palpated and needled at the most tender area to address the SCM pain, which seemed to help resolve the pain although stiffness remained. A press needle was left in place at SJ 5. Her back was still painful at the right SI joint area. The right SI 13 was needled with gentle vibrations for a few seconds and she was asked to move again to reevaluate her discomfort at the low back. This improved her mobility and pain, so a press needle was left at the right SI 13 point.

17. J.S. Male Age: 80

Chief Complaint: Low back/Hip pain

Treatment: Du 17, BL 9, GB 26. SI 13 used as fine tuning after treatment

Patient asked to demonstrate where he feels the pain and which movements which cause the pain.

VEM test is done for herbs.

Patient is side-lying, with painful side up. First, the area of chief complaint is palpated, along the hip, and points are marked with a non-toxic highlighter. All relevant areas are palpated, including jiajis of spine and along Du channel from T 12 down, as well as along Gall Bladder and Bladder channels on sacrum and hip.

Du 17 is needled, and the back and hip are rechecked. One tender spot is left at the left SI joint area, and at the BL 22 area, but all other points, including those on the hip and low back, are released.

BL 9 is used as well as GB 26 (not shown in video) to completely remove remaining tenderness.

After treatment, the patient was asked to stand and do movement again to check for improvement. Some stiffness and tenderness remained at the low back. SI 13 was needled as a support point. Removed after about a minute and a press needle left in place. Counseled to put heating pad on low back.

18. S.E. Male Age: 51

Chief Complaint: Left heel pain and left shoulder pain

Treatment: Du 17, BL 9, HJL5

Begin with palpation of heel and mark tender spots. This is followed by palpation of the shoulder and even mid and low back. The low back is palpated because of the relation to the foot, and the upper back is palpated because it is connected with the shoulder.

Du 17 is needled and the remaining spots which are tender are marked with a different highlighter. BL 9 on the left is needled to address the tenderness at left BL 52 and left GB 30 areas. After needling, it seems that the tenderness at the right side Bladder channel also releases.

Heel pain is remaining after the Essential points. The HTJJ point of L5 on the left is chosen to address this issue. After gentle vibrations of the needle the heel is re-palpated and there is improvement but not completely pain-free. The needle is re-stimulated gently and the heel checked again, and the pain is completely better.

The needles are retained for 20 minutes, with heat lamp on the low back. The patient is asked to move his low back and to notice if the heel pain is better. Since no pain remains, no additional treatment is necessary.

19. B.B. Female Age: 68

Chief Complaint: mid-back pain

Treatment: Du 17, left BL 9

Palpation starts with checking area of chief complaint at BL channels at upper- and mid-back. Du channel is palpated afterwards in this case. Both sides of rib cage are palpated, and left side is found to be tender. Right side below the scapula is also tender.

Treatment begins with Du 17 because T5-T9 were tender from initial palpation. Entire back re-palpated after needling. A few spots left over, one on right side, a few on the left side at mid back and ribs, so the left BL 9 was needled.

She was left for 20 minutes with needles and heat lamp at mid-back.

Final touches not necessary because patient was re-checked after treatment and pain was completely gone.

20. P.M. Male Age: 48

Chief Complaint: Low back pain , SI joint pain

First patient is asked to show movements that cause discomfort.

Treatment: Du 17, right BL 9

Start with palpation of the spine, beginning at around T12-L1 area. Follow with palpation of the Jiaji points, then outer BL channel. If pain clearly shows along Du channel, not necessary to palpate the Jiaji points. Especially in this case, his chief complaint is right along the center at the spine. In other back pain cases, if the pain is more on the sides I might do more investigation of Jiaji points, etc. Important here to check BL points along sacrum. L5-S1 is very tender for him. Du 17 is selected because of tenderness along the Du channel, this is the first step to release before addressing any lateral issues. After needling, back is re-palpated for tenderness and any spots left over are carefully marked. Only spot left over is right sided SI-joint, so I selected BL 9.

Since these two points released all tenderness in the low back, that is the extent of the treatment. Patient is left between 15-20 minutes with a heat lamp on the low back.

After the treatment, patient asked to move again and check for any remaining pain or stiffness. Since nothing left over, no final touches are necessary.

21. C.G. Male Age: 74

Chief complaint: Low back and calf pain

Treatment: Du 17, HJL5, BL 62

Back is palpated along spine and sacrum, marking all tender areas. The calf is also palpated along the BL channel and carefully marked.

Du 17 is needled first because there was tenderness along the lumbar spine. This reduced the pain along the spine and Bladder channel in the low back and thigh. Only a few points remained on the calf along the Bladder channel. For this reason, the Huatuo Jiaji point of L5, on the right, was needled and the remaining tenderness along the calf was eliminated except for at BL 57. BL 62 on the right was added as a support point, which left his calf pain-free.

After 20 minutes with heat lamp on the low back, patient was asked to stand and walk. Since he reported some lingering pain at the calf, I needled the right Huatuo Jiaji of L5 while he was standing and gently vibrated the needle for a few seconds. The needle was then immediately removed and the patient asked to move again, this time the pain was completely gone from the calf.

22. B.G. Female Age: 80

Chief Complaint: Low back pain

Treatment:

Patient palpated while prone, and tender spots were found along the spine and Bladder channel, from the mid-back to the sacrum bilaterally.

Du 17 was needled first, and the back re-checked. Some tenderness remained at the right SI joint and iliac crest and several points at the left SI joint area. The left BL 9 point was needled and the tenderness along the sacrum, on both sides, was released. The only remaining tender spot was along the spine between L4-L5. Du 14 was needled where it was most tender, which resolved the lingering pain at L5.

Needles were retained for 25 minutes and heat lamp applied to the low back.

Since there was no pain after she stood up and moved around, no touch-ups were necessary.

23. G.C. Female Age: 44

Chief Complaint: Neck pain

Treatment: Yin Tang, BL 2, Sp 4, Lr 3, Pc 6

Patient complains of bilateral neck pain and shoulder tension, as well as sinus pressure and tenderness at the jaw at Stomach channel area. She also complained of some bloating and gas, and some constipation, having a bowel movement every other day.

Abdominal tenderness at bilateral ST 27, Ren 12, Pancreas area, Liver/Gallbladder area. All tender spots are carefully marked. Neck palpation revealed tenderness at Trapezius #1, 2, 3, and 4 bilaterally, as well as SCM # 2, 3 and 4 bilaterally.

Acupuncture begins with first reducing tenderness in the abdomen. Yin Tang and bilateral BL 2 were needled, and tenderness remained at the right ST 25 and 27 as well as Ren 12. Sp 4 on the left was used as a support point to address the Ren 12 tenderness, and Lr 3 on the right was used to address the Liver zone on the right around the ribcage. Some tenderness still remained at Ren 12, so Pc 6 on the left was used to support Sp 4. This seemed to relieve the remaining tenderness at Ren 12. At this point I rechecked the neck, which was greatly improved at both the Trapezius and SCM zones bilaterally.

Needles were retained for 20 minutes. After the treatment the patient was asked to re-evaluate the pain in the neck and jaw, which she said had greatly reduced, so there was no need for any final fine-tuning necessary.

*Note: This is a bit of an old video, and I currently don't do things in exactly the same way. For example, in this case I needled BL 2 and Yin Tang at the same time in the beginning, without checking first for improvement in the neck or abdomen. Currently I typically insert one needle at a time, usually starting with Yin Tang, and check for release along the corresponding zone. If necessary I add an additional Essential Point, rather than just doing them all at once in the beginning as seen here. This way I can use fewer needles in the treatment.

24. M.C. Male Age: 70

Chief Complaint: Right side knee pain

Treatment: Yin Tang, BL 2, left Sp 4, right Lr 3

History: diabetes, taking medications and insulin.

First carefully palpate area and mark tender spots along both knees.

Abdomen is then palpated, ST 27 bilaterally is tender, as well as Ren 12, Pancreas zone, Liver zone (under the rib cage and intercostal points of Lr 14 and GB 24, as well as Ren 3-4 area. Groin is also palpated but not found to be tender.

Treatment: Yin Tang, BL2 bilateral to address center line issues, Spleen/Liver zones

Some improvement, but still at liver zone and along upper Ren channel at Spleen/Stomach area

Sp 4 and Lr 3 needled and abdomen re-checked

Improvement at Ren channel and at liver area.

Knees rechecked, tender spots have been reduced there completely.

This is a clear case of knee pain due to internal organ imbalances - Liver and Spleen/Pancreas. After the treatment, recheck once the patient gets up. In this case there was no need for any fine tuning.

A CLINICAL MANUAL OF PRACTICAL ORIENTAL MEDICINE

SAMPLE INTAKE FORM

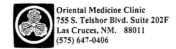

Oriental Medicine Clinic
755 S. Telshor Blvd. Suite 202F
Las Cruces, NM. 88011
(575) 647-0406

Patient's name: _____ ID# _____ DOB: _/_/___ Date __/_/___

Subjective
Chief Complaints: _____
_____
_____
_____

Review of Systems: BODY PAIN SCALE

10	9	8	7	6	5	4	3	2	1
10	9	8	7	6	5	4	3	2	1
10	9	8	7	6	5	4	3	2	1

Temp:_____ Energy:_____

Allergies:_____

GI:_____ Cravings:_____

Sleep:_____ Weight:_____

GU:_____ BP:_____

Emotions:_____

GYN:_____

Objective
Abdominal Palpation: LU (L)(R), PC, HT, ST. LR, GB, PA, SP, LI (L)(R), KI/SI (L)(R) (U)(L), UT, BL, OV/PR(L)(R) ,
          ASIS/IL (L)(R), Groin (L)(R)   Tender Points:_____
Neck Palpation Zone: Trapezius#1 (L)(R), #2 (L)(R) #3 (L)(R),# 4 (L)(R)   _____
          SCM #1 (L)(R), #2 (L)(R), #3 (L)(R), #4 (L)(R)   _____
Back Palpation Zone : Upper(L)(R) Mid (L)(R) Lower (L)(R) Sacrum/ SI Joint (L)(R), Hip (L)(R)
Spinal Palpation: C1, 2, 3, 4, 5, 6, 7, T1, 2, 3, 4, 5, 6, 7, 8, 9, 10, 11, 12, L1, 2, 3, 4, 5, S1, 2, 3, 4, Tailbone

Assessment:_____

Plan:
Position: ☐ Supine ☐ Prone ☐ Side-lying (L)(R) ☐ Sitting down ☐ Standing up
Acupuncture Treatment Minutes:_____ 1ˢᵗ Set: Essential ☐ Yin Tang ☐ BL 2 (L)(R) ☐ Tai Yang (L)(R) ☐ DU 17 ☐ BL 9 (L)(R)
☐ GB12 (L)(R) **2nd Set: Support** ☐ Hutuo Jiaji of L5 (L)(R) ☐ KI 1 (L)(R) ☐ GB25 (L)(R) ☐ GB26 (L)(R) ☐ DU 14 ☐ SI 13 (L)(R)
Synthesis ☐ LU7 (L)(R) ☐ LI4 (L)(R) ☐ ST43/Outer (L)(R) ☐ SP 4 (L)(R) ☐ HT 5 (L)(R) ☐ SI 3 (L)(R) ☐ BL62 (L)(R) ☐ KI 6 (L)(R)
☐ PC 6 (L)(R) ☐ SJ 5 (L)(R) ☐ GB41/42 (L)(R) ☐ LR 3 (L)(R)

_____
_____
_____

☐ Acupuncture Manual ☐ Extended Acupuncture ☐ Infrared Heat (TDP, Foot) ☐ Supplement _____ Weeks/Appt. _____

_____
_____
_____
_____
_____

Signature:_____

CONCLUSION

This book is the conclusion of two years labor. As the saying goes, "persistence pays off" and my dream has come true. Dr. Mateo and I spent hundreds of hours together, asking and answering questions. Without him I could not have done this book, so I am extremely grateful for him. I am very happy and at the same time I am anxious and excited as I look forward to getting the response from those who read this book. The concepts in this book are neither complete nor perfect, but I believe that I have shared the fundamentals of my approach to the treatment of pain.

After reading this book, you might be a little confused given that this system is quite different from what is taught in TCM school. Don't worry about this! I had the same feeling when I began, but after over 10,000 treatments, I now have more confidence in this approach.

I ask you to consider three questions in your daily practice:

What is the patient's body trying to say?

How do their symptoms, complaints, structural balance, internal organs, emotional issues, and stress manifest in their bodies? Listen carefully to the patient to try to discover the source of the problem. It is a new language that we must learn, that of the body, not only verbal communication.

Is this treatment method appropriate for my patients?

Is it comfortable? Does it relieve the patient's pain or help their symptoms improve with each treatment? Is your service accessible and affordable for your patients?

Can I give a better treatment?

Never stop learning. I suggest that you should always be looking at each patient as an individual and learn how to give them the best treatment possible.

I also advise that you try to treat as many patients and conditions as possible, and do your best to get honest feedback in return. Practice makes perfect!

Our job is to make our patients happy with our treatments. If not, we don't often get second chances. Our licenses and titles are meaningless if we don't get results in the clinic.

With every patient I try to put my whole heart and soul into the acupuncture needle.

Thank you for taking the time to read this book.

So, go out and buy #03 needles and start practicing tomorrow, even if you just try using the Essential Points!

This is a very new system that I am just now sharing with others, and I really hope that it will be beneficial to both practitioners and patients. I also hope that this system will continue to develop with the experience of other practitioners, so that it grows, improves, and helps as many people as possible.

I hope that someday we can meet, and learn together. I wish you success in your practice.

November 1, 2013

Masaaki Nakano, DOM

BIBLIOGRAPHY

Xinnong, Cheng. (1987). *Chinese Acupuncture and Moxibustion*. Beijing: Foreign Languages Press.

Kolster, B.C. (2011). *Pictorial Atlas of Acupuncture*. New York: Fullman Publishing.

Matsumoto, Kiiko, and David Euler. (2002). *Kiiko Matsumoto's Clinical Strategies Vol.1*. Massachusetts: Kiiko Matsumoto International.

Matsumoto, Kiiko, and David Euler. (2008). *Kiiko Matsumoto's Clinical Strategies Vol.2*. Massachusetts: Kiiko Matsumoto International.

Miyawaki, Kazuto. (1994).*Yokuwakaru Kikei Chiryo (Ease to understand for the eight extra meridians)*. Tokyo: Taniguchi Shoten.

Ito, Kazunori. (2011). *Yokuwakaru Itami,Chintsu No Kihon To Shikumi (Ease to understand for the pain&analgesic of fundamental&mechanism*. Tokyo: Shuwa System.

Uryu, Ryosuke. (1999). *Shin Kai Igaku (New Comfortable Medicine)*. Tokyo: Tokuma Books.

Gerber, Richard. (2000). *Vibrational Medicine*. (Keiichi Ueno &Tsshirou Manabe, Trans.) Tokyo: Nihon Kyobun sha.

Enomoto, Masaru. (1996*). Hado Towa Nanika(Hado:Tuniing into a new reality)*. Tokyo: PHP Kenkyu jo

Nagata, Kazuya, and Takehito Onose. (2000). *Nou To Kokoro NO Shikumi (Mechanism of the brain and heart)*. Tokyo: Kanki Shuppan.

Sakai, Tatsuo, and Tadashi Hisamitsu. (2011). *Nou NO Jiten (Encyclopedia of the brain)*. Tokyo: Seibido Shuppan.

Nogami, Hruo. (2012). *Nou ,Shinkei NO Shikumi,Hataraki Jiten (Encyclopedia of the brain&nervous about mechanisum&function)*. Tokyo: Sei To Sha.

Shinohara, Shouji. (2000). *Banshin Ryoho(Banshin Therapy)*. Tokyo: Kenkyu Kai.

Kinoshita, Haruto. (1970). *Rinsho Keiketsu Zu(Illustration of Acupuncture Point)*. Tokyo: Ido No Nippon Sha.

Brain Stem. (n.d). In Wikipedia. Retrieved August 20, 2013. http:/en.wikipedia.org/wiki/Brainstem

American Osteopathic Association. (2003) *Foundations for Osteopathic Medicine, 2nd Ed*. R.C. Ward et al. (Eds.) Philadelphia: Lippincott Williams & Wilkins.

AUTHOR'S BIOGRAPHY

1961 Born in Tokyo, Japan

1984 Graduation from Chiba University of Commerce
Bachelor of Business Administration

1990 International Institute of Chinese Medicine Graduation (Santa Fe, NM)

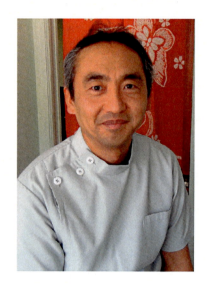

Attended Heilongjiang College of Chinese Medicine (Harbing)

Attended Xi Yuan Hospital – Academy of Traditional Chinese Medicine (Beijing)

Obtained Master of Chinese medicine

NM Licensed Acupuncturist

1991 Opened Oriental Medicine Clinic in Las Cruces, NM

1992 National Certification Commission for Acupuncture and Oriental Medicine (NCCAOM)

NY Licensed Acupuncturist

1993 Doctor of Oriental Medicine (NM)

1995 TX Licensed Acupuncturist

2000 AZ Licensed Acupuncturist
HI Licensed Acupuncturist

Made in the USA
San Bernardino, CA
16 November 2015